Voices of Scleroderma
Volume 1

Voices of Scleroderma
Volume 1

Editors
Judith R. Thompson & Shelley L. Ensz
for the
International Scleroderma Network

ISN Press

Voices of Scleroderma Volume 1, Second Edition

Editors Judith R. Thompson and Shelley L. Ensz
Managing Editor Joanne Grow
Senior Editors Erin Stanley
Production Shelley Ensz
Cover Art Ione Bridgman
Cover Art Assistant Sherrill Knaggs
Distribution Christine Patane

Published by ISN Press 7455 France Avenue South, #266, Edina, MN 55435.

Printed and bound in the United States of America.

Disclaimer: We do not endorse or recommend any treatment for scleroderma or related illnesses. Please consult your doctor or scleroderma expert for treatment advice.

Sources: All personal stories in this book were originally published on the ww.sclero.org website and are reprinted here with written permission of the authors. Pen names have been used when requested and in many instances, author names are different between the website and book stories. All stories have been edited for clarity and content for this book.

Library of Congress Control Number: 2004270838
Publisher: BookSurge, LLC
North Charleston, South Carolina

ISBN: 0-9724623-0-9

Dedication

Lives of great men all remind us
We can make our lives sublime,
And, departing, leave behind us
Footprints on the sands of time.

— Henry Wadsworth Longfellow

From "A Psalm of Life"

To all the great people herein who have left their footprints
on the sands of time and who have let their voices be
heard in the worldwide fight against scleroderma,
"the disease that turns people to stone."

Table of Contents

Chapter 3: Systemic Scleroderma Patient Stories

Systemic Scleroderma

Diffuse Scleroderma

Limited and CREST Scleroderma

Part 2: Juvenile and Localized Scleroderma

Chapter 5: Juvenile Scleroderma

Chapter 6: Localized Scleroderma: Linear and Morphea

Part 3: Autoimmune and Overlap

Chapter 7: Autoimmune Stories

◆❖◆

Acknowledgments

by Judith R. Thompson and Shelley L. Ensz

Judith Thompson is Chair of the Archivist Committee for the International Scleroderma Network (ISN). Shelley Ensz is Founder and President of the International Scleroderma Network, the ISN's Scleroderma from A to Z website at www.sclero.org, and the Scleroderma Webmaster's Association.

This book features over one hundred stories and was created by over one hundred and fifty global volunteers who have worked together via the Internet, cutting across all the barriers of language and politics to share information and support with each other.

All the proceeds of this book series will benefit the nonprofit patient organization, the International Scleroderma Network (ISN).

Certainly, the first credit for this book goes to everyone who has shared their story on ISN's *Scleroderma from A to Z* website where these stories were first posted and where the inspiration for this book was born. These stories are the heart, the soul, and the lifeblood of the website where we all first met and the international nonprofit that we became.

We extend deep gratitude to Professional Network Services of Minneapolis, as they have donated their hosting services, with no limitations, as well as our domain name, and they have faithfully and good-naturedly kept our site going all through the years. In this way, Mike Hastings and Bill and John O'Hanlon have helped to create the cradle where all the personal stories in this book were first shared.

Many thanks go to Arnold Slotkin, a dear friend who calmly insisted that forming the ISN nonprofit would be a fitting outgrowth of the website, despite Shelley's many objections. He gracefully weathered many emails spouting, "Arnold, this is all your fault!" But, of course, it's really to his everlasting credit.

Shelley also extends a hearty thank-you to Judith, for this book and series would not have existed without her enthusiastic urging and leadership. She generously volunteered to archive this series the day after the ISN was publicly launched on January 21, 2002. Within four months she had the original manuscript assembled, which was a mighty task in itself.

ISN board members who have been more heavily involved with the launch of the ISN as well as this book series, in particular, include Gene Ensz and Nolan LaTourelle. ISN legal advisor Linda K. Hopkins of Intelliware International Law Firm provided invaluable advice for this volume.

Ione Bridgman, who is an ISN Artist, painted our wonderful cover design to illustrate our theme of "footprints in the sand" which was then digitally produced by Sherrill Knaggs.

Sonya Detwiler did initial editing and glossary assistance. Story editors for website production for stories in this volume included Judith, Sherry Young, and Kishori Mundargi. A special thank-you goes to Joe Thibault for allowing Julie's story to be shared in Judith's Value of Support introduction to Chapter 4.

Senior editors for this book included Erin Stanley and Joanne Grow. The challenges for the editors were enormous and with each phase, new procedures and editing conventions were established and the manuscript edited once more. We are enormously grateful for their wisdom, skill and persistence in polishing this manuscript.

Professional contributors to this volume included Dr. Joseph H. Korn, Dr. Thomas J. A. Lehman, Dr. Asim Iqbal Qureshi, Gary Barg, and Dr. Magdalena Dziadzio.

Dr. Korn has passed away since the first edition of this book. He was the Alan S. Cohen Professor of Medicine and Rheumatology and Director of the Arthritis Center at Boston University School of Medicine. The center is part of the international Scleroderma Clinical Trials Consortium (SCTC), a group that conducts multicenter trials of therapies for scleroderma. We are forever thankful for Dr. Korn's contribution of the Medical Overview of Scleroderma, which is the medical centerpiece of this volume.

Dr. Lehman specializes in Juvenile Scleroderma, which is the term for any form of scleroderma that begins during childhood. He has written the introduction to our chapter about juvenile scleroderma. He is Chief of the Division of Pediatric Rheumatology for The Hospital for Special Surgery in New York. He is also Professor of Clinical Pediatrics at Cornell University Medical Center.

Dr. Asim Iqbal Qureshi has written a very thoughtful story for this book about Scleroderma and Pregnancy, which discusses the case of an unfortunate fetus. He is with the Department of Obstetrics and Gynecology at the Nishtar Hospital in Multan, Pakistan.

Gary Barg wrote the introduction for our Caregiver section. He is Founder and Editor-In-Chief of Today's Caregiver magazine. He also created caregiver.com and The Sharing Wisdom conference, which brings together caregivers from across the country to share their knowledge and experience as well as honor the annual CareHeroes Awards recipients. His latest book is *The Fearless Caregiver: How to get the best possible care for your loved one and still have a life of your own*, a book with practical advice, poetry and inspirational stories.

Dr. Magdalena Dziadzio is Chair of the Medical Advisory for the ISN. She obtained her medical degree in Poland. She worked in the Department of Internal Medicine at the University of Ancona, Italy. She developed her knowledge about scleroderma working with Prof. Carol Black and her team at the Department of Rheumatology at Royal Free Hospital in London.

Dr. Roy Smith, Kevin Howell, and Dr. Mario Gismondi assisted Dr. Dziadzio with translations for the Italian and Polish stories in this book.

Dr. Roy Smith graduated from the University of Cambridge, England, with a degree in Natural Sciences. He has been working in the field of Medical Electronics. He collaborates with the Royal Free Hospital's Department of Rheumatology, led by Prof. Black, in the area of physiological measurements such as thermography and laser Doppler flowmetry. He assisted in the Polish-to-English translation of Anna's scleroderma story.

Kevin Howell is a Clinical Scientist for Prof. Black at the Royal Free Hospital. He began working in the field of scleroderma in 1991 and uses the techniques of capillaroscopy and infrared thermography. Kevin learned Italian in London and among his friends in Rome.

Dr. Gismondi graduated from the Faculty of Medicine and Surgery at the University of Perugia. He works as a Specialist Registrar in Internal Medicine in the Department of Clinical Medicine at the University of Ancona in Italy. He has given his time to edit the stories written by Italian patients so that he can better understand what it is like to live with this complicated disease.

Other translators for this volume include Dimitra Stafilia who is ISN Greek Translator. She is a qualified translator who works as a project manager in London, and her mother has scleroderma.

Krista Lurtz, ISN Romanian Translator, was the first volunteer to translate our website. She did this when she was very ill and living in Qatar, far away from homeland of Romania. She thereby became the inspiration for the entire international section of the website, which currently includes eighteen languages: Bahasa Malaysia, Chinese, Dutch, English, French,

German, Greek, Hebrew, Hungarian, Italian, Japanese, Kannada, Polish, Portuguese, Romanian, Russian, Spanish, and Turkish.

Please keep in mind that scleroderma affects everyone differently. There is no predictable course for any form of the disease. Nothing in this book is intended as personal medical advice, so please consult your doctor before making any changes to lifestyle or treatments. We do our best to keep the most current information on treatments and clinical trials available on our website.

With so many people involved in this book's production, the only thing for certain is that there are countless people who have played a vital role in its success who are not mentioned here. Many of them are profiled on our website as ISN Representatives or supporters. Some of our volunteers prefer to work anonymously or behind the scenes. Their names deserve to be here also, and they are woven throughout this book in spirit.

We hope it will suffice to say that if you have ever helped the cause of scleroderma in any way, anywhere in the world, you have done a great and grand deed, and we are all very thankful for your footprints in the sand.

Introduction
by Magdalena Dziadzio, M.D., Ph.D.

Dr. Magdalena Dziadzio is Chair of the ISN Medical Advisory. She developed her knowledge about scleroderma working with Prof. Carol Black and her team in the Department of Rheumatology at Royal Free Hospital in London. Dr. Dziadzio also translates the Italian and Polish stories for the ISN's Scleroderma from A to Z website. This introduction is dedicated to Zofia and Stanislaw, Dr. Dziadzio's parents.

Scleroderma is characterised by the transformation of parts of the human body into hard, fibrotic tissue and is, therefore, called "a disease which turns people to stone." It is a rare condition where there is little research, and that is why it belongs to the group of so-called "orphan diseases."

At the moment there is no cure for it and few effective therapies are available. Patients are often left to suffer alone without access to information about their disease. They often wander from hospital to hospital waiting for months or even years for a proper diagnosis.

Every day a physician is expected to solve patients' problems: patients place their trust in the medical system. The reward for a physician taking responsibility for a patient is to cure or to relieve the symptoms. With many diseases success is easy, thanks to modern diagnostic techniques and pharmaceuticals. But when a disease is rare, severe, intractable, and manifests itself in different ways, the physician is faced with a constant battle. Not many doctors are willing to specialise in these orphan diseases. Very little is known, and resources for researchers are scarce. A lot of effort and personal determination is required.

Because scleroderma is rare, it is often not recognised even by medical professionals. This can cause significant delay in diagnosis and once it is made, there are few therapeutic options. Universities and pharmaceutical companies are eager to develop new drug therapies for common diseases, because if these studies are successful the rewards are great: for patients, for scientific understanding and also for commercial profit. However, this does not occur in the scleroderma field. Therefore, there is a need for an international effort to achieve and consolidate progress.

There are, however, some centres where there is substantial research into scleroderma, despite limited resources. Almost every month, new mechanisms in the complicated pathology are discovered. Together with Beirong, David, Chris, and Xu, I spent many hours in the laboratory working with fibroblasts and trying to wring from them the secret of this disease. We hope that one day all those small pieces of information can be put together, allowing us to understand why scleroderma "turns people into stone."

As in any chronic disease, there is necessity of constant contact between patients and their healthcare team. This can be difficult. Many patients do not feel understood, and their symptoms often do not respond well to treatment. Despite this, they try to fight against their disease, and some get stronger and radiate their humanity. Direct contact with patients gives me strength and motivation to continue my work. There is space for friendship to develop. Scleroderma has given me a chance to meet many extraordinary people, both patients and professionals.

Many times I think of Christine, a courageous patient who died of lymphoma. Scleroderma alone was not enough to destroy her. But the disease did not defeat the wonderful love between her and her husband. I remember the wife of Dino, taking care of her husband with love and making sure that everything possible was being done for him. I remember Isabel, asking me for help because she could not breathe. I also keep in mind Elisabeth, who shared with me her happiness of adopting a child. Many other faces, hands, names and surnames tumble through my memory. A porcelain doll from Anita is sitting on my table.

I am honoured to have met extraordinary professionals such as the late Barbara Ansell, who dedicated her life for the children suffering from scleroderma and the late E. Carwile LeRoy, a pioneer in scleroderma research. I take inspiration from many colleagues: Carol, a great rheumatologist who encourages and cares for her patients, who fights for their rights, but away from work, is fragile when confronting their sufferings; Chris, a scientist who, in memory of his mother, chooses to work on this disease rather than to run after professional success; Helen and Rita, two nurses, who every day share the patients' worries and are always ready to listen and to help; and Geraldine, a wonderful woman and physician who teaches future doctors about scleroderma, transmitting her strength and her love.

And finally Shelley Ensz, a most special patient who, using the Internet, told the story of scleroderma and has unified sufferers from many countries, releasing them from their solitude, overcoming the limits of nationality, religion and culture. Her enthusiasm has united an international team of volunteers from all over the world to work together.

Because of these people, the research has to continue, with human contact and the exchange of different experiences. Those who dedicate themselves to work on scleroderma are precious.

My origin and experience let me understand that scleroderma sufferers from the poor or developing countries, like my Poland, are doubly orphaned; there are no specialist scleroderma centres, there is little information, little treatment and no financial support. Therefore, the opportunity given by the Internet is a unique and vital way to provide help for those people. Day after day, the ISN's website at www.sclero.org is growing with new personal stories told by patients and caregivers from all over the world in their own language, enabling these stories to travel across continents.

I am a medical professional as well as scientist who has worked on this disease for almost eight years. I have touched "humans turned into stone," lived their anxiety and despair and, despite the unequal fight against scleroderma, these people make me stronger and I feel useful. I work on the ISN's team of volunteers because I believe that we provide an opportunity for patients to have somebody to contact, someone who can understand their worries and encourage them.

The most important thing is that scleroderma patients do not feel abandoned and are able to see hope on the horizon. Many 'orphan patients' have expressed their gratitude for my work and this is my biggest satisfaction, so I will continue to spread information, advice and hope, along with the many wonderful, talented and dedicated people I am so pleased to be associated with through the International Scleroderma Network.

◆ ❖ ◆

PART 1

Systemic Scleroderma

CHAPTER 1

Systemic Scleroderma
Medical Information

Survival in systemic sclerosis has improved
dramatically over the last two decades, as has
function and well-being among scleroderma patients.

— Dr. Joseph H. Korn

Medical Overview of Scleroderma
by Joseph H. Korn, M.D.

Dr. Korn was the Alan S. Cohen Professor of Medicine and Rheumatology and Director of the Arthritis Center at Boston University School of Medicine in Boston, Massachusetts, USA.

Scleroderma literally means hard skin. That hardness is a result of fibrosis: the formation of scar tissue, which is normal in a healing wound, for example, but is abnormal in fibrotic diseases like scleroderma. While skin changes are the most visible and distinguishing feature of scleroderma, they are far from its only feature. Scleroderma, in its systemic form, is an autoimmune disease, a vascular disorder with injury to blood vessels and abnormal blood vessel function, and a fibrotic or scarring disorder involving multiple organs. Thus, the increased accumulation of collagen and other proteins that occurs in the skin and contributes to its thickening and hardness also occurs in other organs including the lungs, the heart, and the gastrointestinal tract. The relationship among the fibrotic components of the disease, the vascular components of the disease, and the immune and inflammatory events that occur, poses a challenge both for understanding the disease and treating it.

Types of Scleroderma

The term "scleroderma" encompasses two broad categories of disease, each of which may be further subdivided. Localized scleroderma, or morphea, is a localized disorder of skin and, sometimes, the deeper tissues, but it is not a "systemic" disease. It does not involve the internal organs, nor are there the severe blood vessel abnormalities described below for systemic sclerosis or systemic scleroderma.

Localized scleroderma may be characterized by one or several localized skin lesions (often referred to as morphea); widespread skin lesions all over the body (generalized morphea); and linear lesions of thickened skin where the thickness and scarring can spread down to the underlying structures including fat, muscle, and, rarely, even bone (linear scleroderma).

Localized scleroderma may be only a cosmetic problem or may be more serious when the lesions are deep and extensive, and prevent normal motion of joints and inhibit daily activity. Morphea may occur in children in their growing years and, when the involvement extends to deeper tissues, such as in linear scleroderma, growth and development may be affected. Even the cosmetic aspects of localized scleroderma may have important effects on self-image, especially among children.

Systemic sclerosis, as the systemic form of scleroderma is more appropriately called, has widespread effects on the body. Two forms of systemic sclerosis are usually identified: limited cutaneous systemic sclerosis and diffuse cutaneous systemic sclerosis (also called limited and diffuse scleroderma). These two forms of systemic sclerosis are identified by the extent of skin involvement. However, the extent of skin involvement also has important correlates of typical patterns of involvement of internal organs, and, therefore, of ultimate effects on function and mortality. A third form, scleroderma sine scleroderma, is the disease scleroderma but with no thick skin. Although difficult to diagnosis because of the absence of skin involvement, other characteristic disease features clearly put it in the same disease entity.

Limited Cutaneous Systemic Sclerosis

Limited cutaneous systemic sclerosis was once called CREST syndrome, to denote its major features. The letters in CREST stand for **c**alcinosis, **R**aynaud's phenomenon, **e**sophageal dysmotility, **s**clerodactyly and **t**elangiectasia. Calcinosis refers to deposits of calcium in the skin that may be small, even microscopic, or may occasionally be large, lumpy deposits that are readily visible. When widespread they contribute to itching and discomfort in the skin. Larger deposits, particularly when near the surface, may break through the skin and cause sores and drain chronically. Inflammation around deposits of calcium, which is present in the skin as calcium phosphate, may cause pain, particularly when located at sites of pressure, such as the buttocks or elbows. The cause of calcium deposits is not known, and there is no effective treatment to remove them or prevent them; sometimes, surgical removal is needed because of chronic infection or irritation. Some medications, such as colchicine, have been used for the itching caused by calcium deposits and are thought to be helpful, but have not been proven to be effective in clinical trials.

Raynaud's phenomenon is an abnormal response of blood vessels to the cold, most commonly observed in the fingers. On cold exposure, the fingers turn initially pale or white, then blue or purple, and, with re-warming, an intense redness is seen. This triphasic response was described over one hundred years ago by the Frenchman Maurice Raynaud. Raynaud's phenomenon is common in the general population, occurring in as many as ten or twelve percent of individuals. It is more common among women and often shows a familial association. In men, Raynaud's phenomenon sometimes occurs in individuals who work with vibrating instruments, such as chainsaws or jackhammers.

In most individuals in the general population with Raynaud's phenomenon, attacks occur infrequently and only with the extremes of cold exposure. In patients with systemic scleroderma, Raynaud's phenomenon attacks are, in general, more frequent and more severe. Individuals may have multiple attacks a day and, rarely, attacks may last hours or more.

Raynaud's may be complicated by sores at the tips of the fingers known as digital ulcers, due to poor blood supply and impaired healing of cuts and nicks. Repeated episodes may lead to scarring of the tips of the fingers and even progressive loss of finger length. Rarely, gangrene involving the tip of the finger may occur, resulting in more substantial loss.

A number of drugs exist which help to improve blood flow in the fingers, some useful on a chronic basis and others used for acute episodes where there is threatening loss of a finger or part of a finger. Antibiotics are useful in treating complicating infection.

Sympathectomy, the cutting of the supply of nerves that send signals to blood vessels to constrict or clamp down, has been used and may be indicated in some circumstances. This may be a general sympathectomy, involving the interruption of these nerves in the neck, or digital sympathectomy, removing the nerves from the surface of the blood vessels in the fingers. While rarely as severely affected as the fingers, the toes, nose, and ears may also be affected by Raynaud's phenomenon.

Esophageal disease in scleroderma is, initially, a result of the loss of nerve supply to the musculature in the esophagus. This musculature is responsible for the rhythmic contractions of the esophagus, which propel food downward and also prevent the reverse flow of food and other gastric contents, such as acid. In addition, the circular muscles at the very end of the esophagus form a valve or sphincter known as the gastroesophageal sphincter. This valve prevents flow backward from the stomach into the esophagus. Loss of normal muscular function results in both swallowing difficulty (dysphagia) and reverse flow from the stomach into the esophagus (gastroesophageal reflux).

While reflux may, occasionally, occur in almost anyone and is the cause of heartburn (which has nothing to do with the heart), it is a frequent and very troublesome problem in people with systemic sclerosis. Not only does the reflux of the acid cause unpleasant symptoms, but also persistent reflux of stomach acid may cause scarring in the esophagus and actual strictures or blockages that prevent solid foods from passing. When the disease is more advanced, there is replacement of the muscular wall of the esophagus with fibrosis, scar tissue, which further impairs its motility, or contractions.

Whereas in early disease, certain medications may stimulate contractions of the esophagus and help with propelling food downward, once this muscle is replaced by fibrous tissue, such medications are ineffective. Elevation of the head of the bed is useful in helping to keep stomach contents, including acid, in the stomach and preventing reflux into the esophagus. The use of acid-suppressing drugs, particularly the class of drugs known as proton pump inhibitors, has had a dramatic effect in improving symptoms and in preventing scarring of the esophagus.

Sclerodactyly means tight skin on the fingers. Generally, in limited scleroderma or CREST syndrome, tight skin involves only the fingers, toes, and face. Occasionally, after some years of involvement, the hands and the very ends of the forearm may also be involved. By definition, however, involvement of the upper arms, legs, and trunk does not occur in limited scleroderma. Severe involvement of the fingers may lead to contractures, an inability to completely straighten or completely close the fingers. Together with the sometimes-associated digital ulcers, this may cause substantial impairment of hand function. Contractures are caused not only by the thickening of skin on the fingers, but also by the scarring of deeper tissues, such as those surrounding tendons that act as pulleys transmitting muscular contraction to the bones and joints.

Telangiectasia means dilated blood vessels. Sometimes dilated blood vessels are sparse and may be seen on the lips, hands, or chest. Occasionally, telangiectases may be more widespread with extensive large red spots over the face. Sometimes these dilated blood vessels may be viewed at the nail fold where the cuticle meets the base of the nail, using a magnifying lens. Telangiectasia may also occur internally, especially along the gastrointestinal tract. While not usually a problem in limited scleroderma, such telangiectasia in the esophagus, stomach, and intestines may be a cause of low-grade or even substantial bleeding.

While the CREST features of the disease define limited scleroderma, they are not the only types of involvement. Some patients with limited scleroderma develop what is called interstitial lung disease. This is characterized by inflammation in the lungs, which progresses to scarring. In most patients, it is mild and involves only the lower parts of the lungs, but in some patients it may be severe and lead to limited lung function. Another type of lung involvement seen in limited scleroderma is pulmonary hypertension, which is high blood pressure in the blood vessels that lead from the heart to the lungs. One-third or more of patients with limited scleroderma eventuallydevelop some degree of pulmonary hypertension.

In many patients with limited scleroderma, pulmonary hypertension is severe enough to cause major limitation of day-to-day function, and in five percent or more, it may be fatal. Indeed, it is the leading cause of death from scleroderma in patients with limited scleroderma. Recently, new drugs have become available that are effective treatments for pulmonary hypertension and improve lung function. It remains to be seen if their effect is sustained and if their use is able to prolong life.

Diffuse Scleroderma or Diffuse Cutaneous Systemic Sclerosis

As the name implies, patients with diffuse scleroderma have skin involvement that extends all over the body. Characteristically, there is involvement of the trunk, particularly of the chest and abdomen as well as the arms and legs. Skin involvement almost always begins in the fingers and then progresses centrally to involve the forearms, the upper arms and, finally, the trunk. A similar progression is typically seen in the legs. Involvement may range from mild to very severe with very thick, hardened skin that limits mobility.

Involvement of deeper tissues such as tendons, can cause substantial pain in and around joints, and is often mistaken for arthritis. The involvement of structures around tendons can be appreciated by both the patient and the physician as squeaks or rubs around tendons that are often heard or felt best around the wrist and ankles. In addition to impaired mobility, this may also cause pain and discomfort. There may be generalized swelling of the fingers due to inflammation and fluid accumulation, particularly in early diffuse scleroderma. The fluid accumulation is a result of inflammation and should not be treated by diuretics or water pills.

Raynaud's phenomenon occurs in people with diffuse scleroderma, just as it does in people with limited scleroderma. Overall, eighty-five to ninety percent of patients with scleroderma have Raynaud's phenomenon. In people with limited scleroderma, Raynaud's phenomenon is almost always the first symptom and often precedes other aspects of the disease by many years. In diffuse scleroderma, Raynaud's phenomenon often has its onset around the same time as other features of the disease.

Whereas in limited scleroderma, intestinal involvement is usually limited to the esophagus, in diffuse scleroderma the entire gastrointestinal tract, including esophagus, stomach, small intestine, and large intestine may be involved. The underlying problem is similar to that described previously: impaired muscular function leading to impaired motility. Subsequently, scarring of the walls of the bowel contributes to this loss of motility. In the stomach, delayed emptying leads to a sensation of fullness and, consequently, poor food intake. Thickening of the wall of the stomach prevents distention of the wall with food and a sensation of early satiety: feeling full when one has really not eaten very much. Together with delayed gastric emptying, a result of poor peristalsis, early satiety leads people with scleroderma to eat less and have poor nutrition. Impaired motility along the remainder of the gastrointestinal tract contributes to feeling full and the impaired movement of air leads to a chronic feeling of abdominal bloating. Delayed or impaired motility can also lead to overgrowth of bacteria in the small intestine, a place where bacteria do not normally reside, and these bacteria interfere with normal absorption of food. This malabsorption can lead to chronic weight loss and to diarrhea.

There are a number of drugs that improve intestinal motility in scleroderma. Some of these augment the neuroimpulses that are already there, and others directly stimulate the muscles in the wall of the intestines. When there is bacterial overgrowth, antibiotics are useful in improving absorption and in ameliorating the diarrhea and bloating. In the large intestine, the wall of the bowel can become weakened and the large intestine can become very dilated and masquerade as a surgical problem. Surgery in the intestine should be undertaken with great care and only by those aware of intestinal complications of scleroderma.

Lung Involvement

Several types of lung involvement may occur in diffuse scleroderma. Interstitial lung disease, including both inflammation and scarring of the substance of the lung, probably occurs in most patients with scleroderma but is clinically significant in thirty to forty percent. The inflammation interferes with normal exchange of oxygen in the lung and the subsequent scarring destroys normal lung architecture and leads to lung stiffness with an impaired ability to both move air and exchange oxygen. This type of lung involvement occurs most commonly in the first few years of disease and reaches its peak after three or four years. While many believe that treatment with potent drugs that suppress the immune system may be beneficial for this complication, this treatment has not been proven effective, and trials sponsored by the National Institutes of Health (NIH) are currently underway.

Many patients with interstitial lung disease also develop varying degrees of pulmonary hypertension. The combined involvement leads to progressive loss of lung function. Lung disease is the most common cause of death in diffuse scleroderma and its early recognition is important in mounting an effective therapeutic strategy.

In some patients with lung fibrosis, it is thought that chronic aspiration or leak of acid contents of the stomach into the lungs contributes to fibrosis. In addition to involvement of the substance of the lung, some patients with scleroderma develop fluid around the lung sacs, known as pleural effusion. Such collections may become large enough so as to compress the lung and interfere with normal lung function. Drainage of these collections or, in some cases, treatment to prevent their re-accumulation may be helpful.

Heart Involvement

The term scleroderma heart was used years ago to describe the widespread appearance of bands of fibrous tissue, or scarring, throughout the heart of scleroderma patients. Such patches of scar tissue occur even in normal individuals and it is only in younger people with scleroderma that the extent of scarring is clearly excessive. When extensive, such scarring may interfere with normal heart function and muscle contraction. More commonly, when scar tissue involves the electrical pathways of the heart that convey impulses that signal muscle contraction, abnormal rhythms may result. Accumulation of fluid in the sac around the heart, the pericardium, may compress the heart and interfere with its function. This is termed pericardial effusion.

Finally, in patients with pulmonary hypertension, the high pressure in the blood vessels leading to the lungs can result in an overload on the right side of the heart, failure of the right ventricle (which is the chamber that pumps blood to the lungs) causing impaired filling of the heart, and edema (fluid accumulation) in the legs. Such right-sided heart failure is a late sign of pulmonary hypertension and signals a poor outlook.

Kidney Involvement

Kidney involvement was at one time the leading cause of death among patients with diffuse scleroderma. It often appeared suddenly, with the onset of severely high blood pressure, protein in the urine, and associated heart failure. This entity, often called scleroderma renal crisis, is now among the most treatable complications of scleroderma. The key is early recognition of scleroderma renal crisis and early institution of therapy with a class of drugs called angiotensin-converting enzyme inhibitors. These prevent the blood vessel damage that lead to kidney damage and death. It is important for patients with scleroderma to monitor their blood pressure; an elevation in blood pressure accompanies renal crisis in ninety percent of patients. Monitoring the urine for protein is another easy and effective way to check for the appearance of renal involvement in scleroderma.

Muscle Involvement

Muscle inflammation with subsequent muscle destruction is called myositis. Myositis occurs in some patients with scleroderma, particularly those who have overlapping features of systemic lupus erythematosus or dermatomyositis, two illnesses that are related to scleroderma. Muscle inflammation may cause severe weakness and, less commonly, pain. It is effectively treated by corticosteroids (cortisone), often in high doses, and by other drugs that affect the immune system. Myositis may be subtle, with only mild sensation of weakness and fatigue and is often best detected by testing for the presence of elevated muscle enzymes.

Diagnosis of Scleroderma

The diagnosis of scleroderma is a clinical one. In cases where skin involvement is extensive, the diagnosis is easily made. In early disease, where the hands are puffy and the skin is not very thickened, the diagnosis often depends on the recognition of the constellation of symptoms including Raynaud's phenomenon and heartburn, along with physical findings, such as telangiectasia and other blood vessel abnormalities. Sometimes patients with limited scleroderma remain unrecognized for many years because the thickening of the skin on the fingers is not appreciated, and symptoms of heartburn and Raynaud's phenomenon are not associated as due to a single entity.

Laboratory tests are sometimes helpful, especially, in patients with Raynaud's phenomenon, equivocal skin changes, and a paucity of other symptoms. Most patients with scleroderma have antinuclear antibodies, a test that is nonspecific and when abnormal does not necessarily indicate the presence of autoimmune disease. In addition, early in the illness, they may have some features of scleroderma and some features of systemic lupus erythematosus or rheumatoid arthritis. Diagnosis at this early stage may be difficult. Over reliance on laboratory tests may lead to an erroneous diagnosis as often as it leads to the correct one.

The Cause and the Process

The underlying cause of scleroderma is not known. Undoubtedly, genetic factors play a role. Scleroderma patients are more likely to have family members with scleroderma or another autoimmune rheumatic disease, such as lupus erythematosus, than are individuals in the general population. However, this genetic element provides only a predisposition to disease.

Whether enough different genes might lead to disease, or whether some combination of genetic factors and other exposures such as environmental exposures or infections play a role, is as yet unknown.

Some data suggest that exposure to industrial solvents may predispose to scleroderma in some patients. These studies require confirmation. There are apparent clusters of disease, increased numbers of cases in small communities, which suggest an environmental agent may play a contributing role. In addition, scleroderma-like syndromes have been clearly linked to agents as varied as contaminated rapeseed oil (used for cooking in Spain), polyvinylchloride monomer (in industrial workers), and a contaminant in L-tryptophan, which was used as a food supplement. These 'accidents' at least suggest that scleroderma might be caused or triggered by environmental agents in a susceptible individual.

Whatever the trigger or triggers, several processes ensue. The earliest events involve the immune system and the blood vessels. Blood vessel involvement is typified by Raynaud's phenomenon, which starts as an abnormal reaction of blood vessels to the cold, but goes on to structural damage of vessels, which become occluded by scar tissue. This is likely initiated by damage to the inner lining of the vessel, the endothelium, a damage whose cause is unknown.

The second early series of events are immunological. The involvement of the immune system is evidenced by the presence of antinuclear antibodies, which are antibodies to components of the nuclei of cells. Such antibodies are seen in a number of autoimmune diseases including systemic lupus erythematosus and polymyositis. There is also evidence of the disease in activation of T cells and monocytes, which are critical cells in the immune system. Clearly, these cells are responsible for causing inflammation, damage, and subsequent scarring in the lungs.

Initially at least, the scarring or fibrosis seen in scleroderma is a result of inflammation. Factors released by immune cells called cytokines are known to stimulate scar formation. Damaged blood vessels also release such cytokines, which turn on fibroblasts of the skin and elsewhere to make increased amounts of collagen and other connective tissue proteins, which form scar tissue.

Eventually, however, it appears that fibroblasts in the skin and elsewhere become independent of stimulation and continue to make excessive amounts of scar tissue on their own. Thus, the scarring lesions in the skin, lungs, and even in the blood vessels may become an autonomous event; that is, an event that is independent of further abnormalities in the immune system or further blood vessel damage.

Treatment

Like most other diseases, excepting infections and some tumors, scleroderma is an incurable disease. Incurable, however, does not mean untreatable. There are effective treatments for muscle inflammation, blood vessel disease, intestinal motility and, of course, for kidney disease.

There is active investigation into new treatments for skin disease, an area where no treatment has ever been proven to be effective. These new treatments target cytokines, those messengers that stimulate fibroblasts to make increased amounts of collagen, the bedrock of fibrosis.

Other new treatments are directed at improving blood vessel function both by dilating blood vessels and replacing substances lost by damaged blood vessels that help promote blood flow.

It is very likely that over the coming decade, more effective treatments for both the vascular disease and the fibrosis of scleroderma will be forthcoming. In any case, patients with scleroderma should be optimistic. Survival in the disease has improved dramatically over the last two decades, as has function and well-being among scleroderma patients. It can still be a devastating disease, but with cooperation among patients and physician, the outlook has become much better.

Scleroderma and Pregnancy
by Asim Iqbal Qureshi, M.B.B.S., F.C.P.S.

Dr. Asim Iqbal Qureshi is with the Department of Obstetrics and Gynecology at Nishtar Hospital in Multan, Pakistan.

The Case of the Misfortunate Fetus

Khalida was a thirty-three-year-old housewife married to Akram, a thirty-five-year-old factory worker. They were married for nine years and were well settled in a small town of Pakistan. The couple had been trying to achieve pregnancy, but had failed to do so. They never sought any medical advice; rather they left it to God's will.

Over the last six years, she was not feeling very well and used to get fatigued very easily and, occasionally, had heartburn and acidity. She sometimes visited a local physician, but he was only providing her palliative care with vitamins, tonics and antacids. In addition, she noticed that her skin was not as soft as it used to be some years back, but she never gave any importance to this change. Nobody was aware of the fact that Khalida was developing scleroderma.

Time went by and, suddenly, there was a magnificent stroke of luck for both Khalida and Akram when Khalida was found to be pregnant while evaluating her for her missed periods. It was a time of great joy for the entire family. She got booked in an antenatal clinic, and during the routine investigation, it was found that she was passing a small amount of proteins in her urine. She was referred to a specialty clinic and there her diagnosis of scleroderma was made for the very first time.

Her physicians and obstetrician were worried about the course of the disease and its impact on her pregnancy. Although both Khalida and Akram were briefed about the scleroderma and its possible course, they did not try to understand anything except that she was pregnant with a fetus of sixteen weeks of age who was, otherwise, doing fine so far.

Her antenatal visits were planned more frequently to closely monitor her pregnancy and the course of scleroderma. Initially, she was enthusiastic about attending the antenatal clinics, but after two or three visits, her attendance at the antenatal clinics became poor. She even ignored the advice to visit the medical specialists.

She made her next antenatal visit after missing four consecutive appointments and by that time, her pregnancy had progressed to twenty-nine weeks. That day she had a severe headache and her blood pressure was remarkably high. Urine tests revealed that she was passing large amounts of proteins. She was strongly advised for urgent hospitalization, but she disappeared again. A week later, she came back complaining of loss of fetal movements. Still she had very high blood pressure. Blood tests revealed that her kidneys were not functioning properly and the ultrasound scan revealed that the fetus was dead in her womb. It was really a difficult time for both Khalida and Akram to go through this tragedy. She was admitted in the labor ward. After stabilization of her blood pressure, the labor was induced and after twelve hours, a dead male baby was delivered. The baby was, otherwise, normal in appearance except that there were no signs of life. For the follow up, she was referred to medical specialists, but unfortunately; she never returned for the follow up. It was tragic that Khalida lost her baby, not because of any congenital abnormality or birth defect, but due to the complications provoked by the scleroderma.

Comments

Scleroderma is a rare, chronic autoimmune disease, which includes a heterogeneous group of limited and systemic conditions causing hardening of skin and certain internal organs. Systemic sclerosis implies involvement of both skin and other sites, particularly, certain internal organs.

Each year five to twelve new cases of Systemic sclerosis are diagnosed per million in the population. It primarily affects females who are thirty to fifty years old at onset and the ratio of women to men is about four to one. Because of the rare occurrence in humans and non-availability of suitable animal models, there is very limited understanding about this disease at the moment.

The cause of scleroderma is unknown. Some cases of scleroderma have been linked to chemical exposures. Genetics, fetal cells, and viruses might also be factors in the development of scleroderma. At present, there are no proven treatments or cure for any form of scleroderma. However, there are effective therapies for many of the symptoms.

The occurrence of scleroderma and pregnancy is even more rare, so no reliable data of statistical significance is available pertaining to the incidence or outcome for either the mother or the fetus. It is possible that a patient with scleroderma can achieve pregnancy, although the ability to get pregnant may be less.

Previously, the miscarriage rate was considered to be high; however, recent studies show no increase in the miscarriage rate among the patients with scleroderma. Pregnancy may adversely affect the course of the systemic form of scleroderma (systemic sclerosis) with renal disease being a particular and lethal risk.

The second half of pregnancy term is a dangerous period with the risks of rapidly developing high blood pressure and kidney failure as well as the interruption of pregnancy, as it happened in the case of Khalida.

Ideally, the woman with scleroderma should seek advice before planning a pregnancy. If there is evidence of severe kidney disease, pulmonary hypertension (high blood pressure in the blood vessels of lungs) or myocardial fibrosis (damaged heart muscle), a therapeutic abortion should be offered in the best interest of maternal health. If the patient chooses to proceed with the pregnancy, antenatal examinations should be more frequent. Careful assessment of blood pressure, heart, lung and kidney function should be done at each antenatal visit. Symptomatic treatment and appropriate nutritional supplements should be provided to the patient.

Delivery should be conducted in a well-equipped labour room with readily available intensive care facilities because such a patient may collapse during or shortly after labour. By virtue of the nature of disease, scleroderma may pose problems for the anaesthetist to administer anaesthesia or pain relief during labour. Regardless of the type of anaesthesia and whether delivery is by the vaginal route or Caesarean section, an experienced anaesthetist should be aware of the disease status of patient.

The post-natal period should be monitored carefully as high blood pressure with kidney and heart failure may occur even after the baby is born.

◆ ❖ ◆

Systemic Scleroderma Symptom Checklist

Please consult your doctor if you have two or more of the following symptoms, which are sometimes due to systemic sclerosis (scleroderma). Systemic scleroderma may disqualify a person for life and/or health insurance in some countries. Sometimes certain lab work or biopsy results may force an unwelcome diagnosis into the medical record.

Circulation
❑ Swelling of hands, feet and/or face
❑ Raynaud's: fingers and/or toes turn white or blue due to cold or stress
❑ Ulcers (sores) on fingertips or toes

Gastrointestinal
❑ Difficulty swallowing
❑ Heartburn (reflux)
❑ Constipation, diarrhea, irritable bowel syndrome

Heart, Lungs, Kidneys
❑ Shortness of breath
❑ Pulmonary (lung) fibrosis
❑ Aspiration pneumonia
❑ Pulmonary hypertension
❑ High blood pressure or kidney (renal) failure
❑ Right-sided heart failure

Muscles & Tendons
❑ Tendonitis, or carpal tunnel syndrome
❑ Muscle aches, weakness, joint pain

Excessive Dryness or Sjögren's Syndrome
❑ Excessive dryness of the mucus membranes (such as eyes, mouth, vagina), which is sometimes called Sjögren's Syndrome

Skin
❑ Tight skin, often on hands or face
❑ Calcinosis (calcium deposits)
❑ Telangiectasia (red dots on the hands or face)
❑ Mouth becomes smaller, lips develop deep grooves, eating and dental care become difficult

Many of these symptoms can occur by themselves or can be due to other things. Symptoms such as heartburn, high blood pressure, constipation, and muscle aches are very common in the general population. More unusual symptoms, such as tight skin and/or pulmonary fibrosis, may be more likely to lead to a scleroderma diagnosis.

◆ ❖ ◆

CHAPTER 2

Systemic Scleroderma
Caregiver Stories

I wish all the people suffering from scleroderma to be able to manage to live in a decent manner, without having to put up with this terrible suffering and other things that the disease, unfortunately, brings.

— Antonio Sabino

Introduction to Caregiving
by Gary Barg

Gary Barg is Founder and Editor-In-Chief of Today's Caregiver magazine. He is also creator of CAREGIVER.COM and the Sharing Wisdom conference. His latest caregiving tool is The Fearless Caregiver: How to Get the Best Possible Care for Your Loved One and Still Have a Life of Your Own.

Over the past few years, I have been blessed to spend time traveling the country talking to my favorite people in the world—family and professional caregivers. I have spoken in rural towns at country health fairs and at annual national conferences. So many of the caregivers I have met along the way are forever etched in my mind, as are many of the events. But truly some occasions are more memorable than others.

In 1999, I was honored to speak at a national scleroderma conference and I have to say, that is one event that I will never forget. Not necessarily because of the locale, although I love San Diego, rather, I will always remember that event because it was the first time a session audience took my words so very much to heart. I always start my sessions giving notice that I don't want to only hear my voice during the following hour. These sessions should be a true interaction between everyone involved. Once we got started, this particular session turned into an extremely lively support group. The hour was filled with people openly sharing the tips, techniques and advice that helped them as they were caring for their loved ones who were living with scleroderma. The feeling of warmth and willingness to share with one another that permeated the room was exhilarating and I continue to refer to that day in many of the seminars I've presented in the ensuing years. For you see in caregiving, giving is truly the same as receiving.

We named our annual caregiving conference "Sharing Wisdom," because that's what successful caregiving is all about, finding wisdom through the professionals who lead the sessions as well as the sponsors and service providers, but most importantly, finding wisdom from one another.

When I first started in my personal journey as a family caregiver, other family caregivers would stop me as I walked into adult living facilities or hospital waiting rooms asking for my advice. At first, I thought it was kind of neat that I maybe looked like a doctor or even someone in the know, until I began to realize that we were all asking for help from anyone we ran into. We shared whatever wisdom we happened to have and were rewarded, equally, in return.

To take the best advantage of the time spent in doctor's offices, waiting rooms or at seminars and conferences, introduce yourself to your fellow caregivers and take a moment to see what you have in common and what you can teach each other. You will be astonished at how much you learn and how much you share.

The Road Less Traveled by M. Scott Peck is one of my favorite books, mainly because of the first line in the book: "Life is difficult." Once I read those three little words, I got my money's worth without going any further. Except I would go further by saying that a caregiver's life is exceptionally difficult. I cannot imagine a single caregiver who does not wish things were different and why not. Look at the statistics.

Presently, on average, a caregiver will be responsible for the directed expenditures of forty thousand dollars a year caring for their loved one. Out-of-pocket, he or she will spend almost ten percent of their annual salary. Caregivers will lose over six hundred thousand dollars in opportunities and promotions during the lifetime of his or her career and over sixty-three percent will consider depression to be his or her most commonly felt emotion.

Then why do we do it? Because we can't *not* do it; because our loved ones need us; because we never even asked ourselves if there were any other way; and because it is who we are. So now what? How do we go from being mother; father; sister; brother; lover; spouse or dedicated daughter to being the dietitian; therapist; insurance specialist; immediate medical expert; chauffeur, psychologist and pharmacist as our caregiving role demands? And how do we keep our relationship with our loved ones, families, friends and neighbors, not to mention our jobs, which a third of us end up losing?

I firmly believe the way that we achieve all of our goals as caregivers is by actually taking on a new job role. The role is one I call being a Fearless Caregiver. A Fearless Caregiver is a caregiver who understands that they have a job to do as a full member of their loved one's care team. No less important than the case manager, therapist or even the doctor. All team members have jobs to do, yours is to learn all you can about your loved one's situation and to act as his or her advocate.

You are there not only to represent your loved one, but also to present a human face to those within the healthcare system. Yours is a crucial role. No matter how much they care, your doctor sees at least twenty-five patients a day, your case manager and therapist have larger case loads than ever and other members of a hospital or care facilities team probably have never even laid eyes on your loved one.

Over the years as publishers of Today's Caregiver magazine and as caregivers ourselves, we have spoken with thousands of other caregivers, and one thing has become crystal clear. A caregiver can be heard in today's healthcare system. And we can be heard. We have found significant common traits among the caregivers who are being heard. First, they believe they can make a difference. Second, they understand that the role they plays in a loved one's care is just as important as the role of any of the professional caregivers. And third, they ask questions. They ask lots of questions. They research and do not easily take "no" for an answer. They become a Fearless Caregiver.

Fearless Caregivers knows their rights concerning his or her loved one's insurance plan, and are able to exercise those rights. A Fearless Caregiver knows how to find the latest treatment options and present qualified research to the members of their loved one's care team. A Fearless Caregiver IS a member of their loved one's care team.

But do you know what the very first step to such care is? It's caring for you. I know, I know, I hear you saying, "Who has time to care for me? I spend all my time caring for him (or her)." My answer to that is, who will care for you and your loved one when you take ill due to exhaustion or from simply not caring for yourself?

You cannot go through caregiving unchanged. Nobody can. My wish for you as caregivers is that caregiving allows you to achieve an inner strength that you may never have thought you could possess. The way to get to that place is to become acutely aware of your position and your power as your loved one's caregiver.

I urge you to take the time to carefully read every story in this book. The professional and family caregivers who share their stories are your teachers as you are theirs. I believe it is an essential tool for anyone who loves someone living with scleroderma.

◆❖◆

Amy Fogarty
Father, Systemic Sclerosis
Illinois, USA

This was written for a speech that I delivered to my Communications class.

Imagine for me, if you would, that in certain areas of your body the skin has begun to thicken and harden. Then on top of this, you have a painful sensitivity to cold, frequent heartburn, stiff joints and various other internal problems.

These are the things that my father has to deal with daily due to a rare disease known as scleroderma, which, when literally translated, means the hardening of the skin. I'm here today to inform you of some of the facts surrounding scleroderma, the types of scleroderma and the support groups affiliated with scleroderma.

Scleroderma is a chronic autoimmune disease of the connective tissue. Generally, it is classified as a rheumatic disease that, in the systemic form, affects an estimated eighty thousand to one hundred thousand people in the United States.

If one were to count the number of people with Raynaud's phenomenon (which I'll tell you about later) and at least one symptom of scleroderma, the count would reach nearly one hundred and fifty thousand, and there are even more carrying the localized form of the disease.

Overall, female patients outnumber the men, four to one. The average age of diagnosis is in the forties, although there are many exceptions in scleroderma as it is found not only in children, but also in elderly patients.

The exact cause of scleroderma is unknown, but doctors have found that scleroderma involves an overproduction of collagen. Depending on the form of scleroderma, the effects may either be visible to the open eye, or invisible and only seen internally.

Scleroderma is a highly individualized disease with symptoms that may range anywhere from mild to potentially life-threatening. There is no cure for this disease, but there are many treatments for those afflicted. While the bad aspects of scleroderma definitely outweigh the good, scleroderma is not contagious, cancerous or malignant, or inherited, generally speaking.

There are two different types of scleroderma: localized and systemic. Systemic sclerosis is the more common and deadly form of scleroderma in which the immune system damages two main body areas; the small blood vessels and the collagen-producing cells located in the skin and throughout the body.

These areas include the connective tissue in many parts of the body such as the skin, esophagus, gastrointestinal tract, lungs, kidneys, and heart. They also may include the muscles and joints in the body.

There are many effects of this form of scleroderma. First and foremost, nearly all scleroderma patients are cold sensitive. This is a result of the blood vessels in the fingers narrowing and sometimes, completely closing off the channel of blood in the fingers. This often causes small cuts on the hands to heal very slowly. Because of this decreased blood supply, the majority of scleroderma patients are also very sensitive to cold temperatures.

This vascular part of the disease is the cause of Raynaud's phenomenon that afflicts approximately ninety percent of those with systemic sclerosis. Raynaud's phenomenon causes fingers to change color with exposure to cold temperatures.

The overproduction of collagen is the part of scleroderma that causes the thick and tight skin, lung problems, gastrointestinal problems, and the heart problems associated with this form of the disease. When a body is functioning normally, the immune system sends out signals to the collagen producing cells to form a scar after an injury or infection has been cleared. When one has scleroderma, scar tissue is produced, for no apparent reason, and simply builds on the skin and other internal organs.

Systemic sclerosis can also be divided into two categories known as limited and diffuse. These two categories refer to the amount of skin involvement. While both forms produce internal organ damage, the limited form has a tendency to be less severe.

The limited form is often referred to as the CREST form. CREST stands for calcinosis, or calcium deposits in the skin; Raynaud's phenomenon, which I discussed earlier; esophageal dysfunction, or acid in the esophagus felt as heartburn; sclerodactyly, the thick and tight skin of the fingers; and telangiectases, a particular type of red spots that may appear on the skin.

Localized scleroderma, more commonly affects children. This type of scleroderma is usually only found in a few places on the skin or in the muscles. While this form of scleroderma does not affect any internal organs, it is based in the collagen-producing cells in some areas of the skin instead of affecting all areas. This form is confined to a local area of skin and tissue.

Localized scleroderma is generally associated with thick patches of skin, morphea, or with linear scleroderma, which is a line of thickened skin that extends down one of the extremities. This type of scleroderma rarely, if ever, develops into systemic sclerosis.

If you, a family member, or a friend has scleroderma, there are many support groups available to help one deal with the emotional effects of this disease. The www.sclero.org website provides links to other websites affiliated with scleroderma and stories of patients as they tell of their connection with the disease as well as many facts that may help people understand this rare disease.

A few years ago, Bob Saget, from *America's Funniest Home Videos*, made a television movie called *For Hope* as a tribute to his sister who died of scleroderma. I saw this movie when it came out, though it was before my father had been diagnosed. I think that if you'd like to get a first-hand look at what scleroderma can do, this would be a worthwhile movie to obtain.

In conclusion, I hope that I've helped you understand a little more about this disease. You should know, however, that not all patients suffer as horribly as I may have made it sound. The affects of scleroderma may vary from patient to patient.

If more people were made aware of this disease, maybe more support would be given to the research involved in finding a cure for those afflicted. Remember this: though it is not a widespread disease that you will read about in the media, it still affects hundreds of thousands daily. Diagnosed in 1995, I've watched my father deal with the affects of this disease daily, never knowing what the outcome is going to be.

◆ ❖ ◆

Antoinette "Toni" Sutton
Husband Jeff, Stem Cell Transplant
Michigan, USA

On November 1, 1999, my husband, Jeff, was diagnosed with scleroderma and our life changed, as we knew it. We had a seven-month-old son and had been married just over two years.

Jeff was just twenty-three years old and had been seeing doctors for over a year trying to find out why he was having symptoms such as his hands and feet turning a blackish color in cold temperatures as well as having terrible pain throughout his body every day. When his family doctor sent him to University of Michigan for further diagnosis, that is where our journey with scleroderma began.

We were told that Jeff had a very fast progression of the disease. The skin on his arms, legs, chest and back were already tightening. He also was affected in his stomach and throat, which gave him acid reflux problems, and showed signs of damage to his lungs (though minimal). Jeff lost approximately forty pounds in a matter of a few months and could not even drink a sip of water without pain in his chest.

On the day Jeff was diagnosed, he was told to go home and quit his job as a cabinet builder and finisher, and that he had approximately five years before the disease could possibly kill him. As you can imagine, this felt like someone just hit our family with a truck. How could this happen to us? Well, we met the people that I say saved my husband's life.

The doctors at the University of Michigan worked very hard to present us with all of the options, and Jeff was offered a chance to participate in the stem cell transplant research program. After reviewing all our choices, we realized that this was our only option to have a chance at spending our life together as we had planned.

On March 3, 2000, after many tests and a lot of hospital visits, Jeff was administered the stem cells that were going to change our lives. I am happy to say that Jeff is now seventeen months past his transplant and to look at him, you would never know he was sick. He is working full time and living his life as he had always planned.

We are very grateful that we were given the opportunity to take part in the stem cell research and that it was successful. Now my two-year-old son can play with his dad and enjoy it!

I would recommend that anyone who thinks that they may have this disease seek out a rheumatologist and have the tests done. There is hope and the more people who know about it, the better.

Antonio Sabino
Mother, Progressive Systemic Sclerosis
Italy

I am writing this story on behalf of my mother, Gianna, who is not very good at using a computer. Her disease was diagnosed in May 1998, but the symptoms were already present a long time before that. Her hands were affected at the very beginning as they no longer had the same elasticity and started to become white, cold and, above all, stiff in their movement.

Then the disease extended to other parts of the body, always involving the skin, with the formation of lesions and hardening of the skin. Afterwards, she developed other classic manifestations of the disease, including gastroesophageal reflux and widespread pain, which have required a special diet as well as the use of numerous drugs like steroids.

Currently, my mother is seen regularly at the Department of Rheumatology in the University Clinic in Padua. Over and above the classic symptoms of the disease, she now also has renal problems due to scleroderma. She suffers from recurrent bouts of gastric reflux, mostly at night, that cause her terrible pain, and she also has fever associated with breathing difficulties as well as a very intense feeling of abdominal bloating. Furthermore, there is a hardening of her skin to such an extent that taking blood is hardly possible, together with a loss of strength and general fatigue.

At this point, I'll stop because maybe I cannot be precise enough, but in less than two years, my mother's life has totally changed for the worse, really the worse. Then reading the letters published on www.sclero.org from other people, I found out that their symptoms and medications are the same as hers.

So if any of you would like to get in touch with her, possibly to meet, or just to talk, with the intention of improving the situation for those who find themselves having to fight this strange and awful disease, I would be happy to put you in contact. We are hopeful of finding someone with whom we can try to overcome the problems created by this disease and by its medications.

Thank you for your attention. I wish all the people suffering from scleroderma to be able to manage to live in a decent manner, without having to put up with this terrible suffering and other things that the disease, unfortunately, brings.

◆ ❖ ◆

Dimitra Stafilia
Mother, Scleroderma
Greece

Dimitra Stafilia is the ISN's Greek Translator. Below is her story in English. This story is also available in Greek in Chapter 9.

My mum has been suffering from scleroderma since 1992. It first started as an acute pain in her fingers. Whenever it was cold, her fingers would turn blue and then white. She first went to an angiologist, who suspected that the problem could be more serious and referred her to a rheumatologist, who diagnosed her as suffering from scleroderma. At least she was lucky enough to have doctors willing to examine all possible explanations for her disease.

That was a new reality for the whole family. We had no idea what it was, where it came from and how serious it was. I was still in high school and had no concept of the suffering it would cause her. Admittedly, my mum started reading and learning about her disease. The use of the Internet was not that widespread in Greece, so she mainly got her information from encyclopedias and from my aunt in New York.

Where did her disease come from? I have read articles that say that it could be environmental or genetic. For many years, we lived within an industrial zone. My father, until his retirement four years ago, worked for a company that produces nickel. Actually, it produced a mixture of iron and nickel. The soil that was mined also included small quantities of cobalt and copper. I have not heard of any other people living in the area having scleroderma, but then again, we stayed in the area longer than most of them did.

Over the years her illness progressed rather badly. She got arthritis and her fingers were disfigured; the nails split so that you could see the flesh beneath them. She got pulmonary fibrosis; problems with her esophagus; high blood pressure and dyspnea (shortness of breath), just to name a few of the problems. She has to take a cocktail of drugs to fight the individual symptoms and visit specialist doctors regularly to run tests for her heart and lung conditions. The use of cortisone for the fibrosis caused her osteoporosis (still at the initial stage). Because of the drugs she is also overweight. This worsens her condition. My mother is fifty-one years old.

I started looking into her disease when I went to University. I visited the Royal Free Hospital in London and I wrote to the American scleroderma association. However, there was no documentation I could get hold of easily in Greek, and there was no way to know whether her doctor was in touch with the latest developments or whether he performed the necessary tests.

I believe that the patient should be able to know about, question and agree on the treatment, and this was not happening in my mum's case. Thus began my interest in translating the pages of the ISN's website, to give other Greek patients the opportunity to know a little bit more and to know that there are other people with similar problems.

As for myself, I am a qualified translator working as a project manager in London who thinks that any academic or professional achievement is not enough, as I am not around to support my mother psychologically. So this is my small contribution.

Elizabeth Alvarado
Husband, Systemic Scleroderma
Arizona, USA

My husband was diagnosed in July 2000. We didn't expect to hear he had scleroderma, and at first, neither of us understood what it was. His doctor had run a lot of tests and given him medicine to take. There were so many pills, but none of them worked.

We were finally sent to a specialist, who sat us down and gave us the news that would change our life forever. My husband and I were in shock and couldn't speak a word. My husband has always been very healthy throughout his life. He played in sports in high school and was always very active.

After we left the doctor's office, we both just sat in the car and cried and cried; the tears just kept coming. He is a good man who doesn't deserve what was to change his life forever. He's a great father of two teenagers, a hard worker, and great husband. I know no one deserves to have scleroderma.

We had decided not to tell our kids until the time was right. We got home and right away my daughter asked, "What does daddy have?"

I just started to cry all over again, so we had to sit both of them down and tell them. They were so upset and didn't understand what it was or why it happened to their daddy. Our son, who is the strong-minded child, was in tears. He told my husband that he would help him in any way he could.

My husband and son were always playing catch with the football, but now he can't do that because his hands are always in pain. I know that there is no cure, but I pray each day that a cure will be discovered.

My husband is very young, only thirty-six years old, and scleroderma doesn't run in his family. Well, now we take each day at a time. We have our love for one another to beat this and win!

◆ ❖ ◆

John T.
Mother-in-Law, Systemic Scleroderma
Canada

My mother-in-law found out that she has systemic scleroderma a number of years ago. She has been progressing downward. She since has been admitted to the intensive care unit (ICU) for a heart attack.

She had worked as a custodian for a number of years, and that may be a factor in causing her scleroderma as she had worked with and had been exposed to a number of chemicals that had possibly brought on the scleroderma. Has anyone else out there been a custodian and now suffers this affliction?

Nicole Shields
Father, Systemic Scleroderma
Missouri, USA

I am eighteen years old and my father has systemic scleroderma. He has had this disease for about two years now.

I'm not sure why my father has to suffer through so much pain, and I pray every day that he will be relieved from his pain. I remember being so scared of losing my father. He is one of the greatest men in the world. He's more compassionate and wiser than anyone else I have ever come across. I lost my mother when I was two years old and I really was scared of losing my father, also. I have a stepmother whom I love more than anything. She pretty much raised me. I also have two younger sisters, one seven and one thirteen, and two older brothers, one twenty-nine and one twenty-seven.

I remember one day, my youngest sister wanting to sit up on my dad's lap, and she was quite the chunk for her age. Anyway, my dad tried to lift her up and he couldn't. His joints hurt too badly. I sat there and watched him tell my baby sister that he couldn't hold her right then because, "It hurts too much." That broke my heart. But this winter, it's not that bad. His skin is loosening up and he can go outside and do yard work and he can put my little sister on his lap.

And this next summer, he'll be able to walk me down the aisle when I get married. I have wanted that since I was a little girl, but even more so since he got sick. I really believe that my father is healing. He gets stronger every day and can do more and more. I just wanted to let everyone know, that it may seem like a long time before you get well, but with enough prayer and hope, everything will be okay.

◆ ❖ ◆

Patricia McDonald
Husband, Diffuse Scleroderma
Canada

My husband was diagnosed with limited scleroderma in June of 2000. We had never heard of the disease before, but we know a lot now, thanks to www.sclero.org.

It all started when his hands began to swell, and then painful ulcers began to form on the ends of his fingers. His skin is hard and thick. It has started around his eyes, and the back of his neck is itchy and burns. He also has arthritis, which bothers him a lot. The cold drives him crazy, and it takes quite awhile to warm up again.

Lately, he has been having problems breathing and soreness in the chest. He had a breathing test done a month and a half ago, and it was all right. He is now going for a CT scan, dye tests and a swallowing test for the esophagus.

We will be going to Baltimore in September to see Dr. Wigley. I will update more on my husband's condition when we return from Baltimore.

Update

My husband was diagnosed with diffuse scleroderma this time, although right now the doctor says there is no internal involvement so far.

The scope of the esophagus showed some abnormalities, but there is no heartburn yet and no difficulty swallowing. The arthritis is bothering him a lot, his appetite is not very good, and he has lost fifteen pounds since he has been diagnosed.

Dr. Wigley is the best doctor that we have spoken to so far. He explained this disease in a very understanding way and took a lot of time talking with us. He mentioned a study test that is being done on the lungs that will determine how soon or how long it will be before internal involvement occurs.

We live in Canada, so it is quite a distance to keep in contact with Dr. Wigley, and he was so kind as to give me his email address. We will keep him updated with my husband's condition through email.

From what I have read about diffuse, it is just a matter of time and internal involvement will occur, so this was very scary to hear. Does anyone know how long it takes before it goes internally? What can I do to help my husband?

I am very worried about him, but I have to put up a good front, so he doesn't get too upset. Lying in bed at night is my worst time; this is where I have my crying sessions. We have only been married one year, and I wonder how many more we will have, before this terrible disease takes him away from me.

Update – May 2001

Since my last update, my husband has had cataract surgery on both eyes. He was having heartburn, but it is under control with medication. He has lost a lot more weight. He will have a gastroscopy, which is an examination of the throat (esophagus), stomach, and part of the small intestine (duodenum).

The cords in his arms keep him awake at night. They are very painful, because the skin is so tight and hard. His fingers are starting to curl quite badly, which makes it hard for him to do things, like brush his teeth, hold a bar of soap, put on shaving cream, peel vegetables, hold onto his pills, and pick small things off the floor.

He is now on Workers' Compensation, because he was exposed to silica dust. He worked at painting and sandblasting for twenty years, and it is considered a work-related disease. There have been a lot of changes in my husband's health over the past year. I only wish I could take away some of the pain he endures.

Srikanth "Jonty" Manam
Mother, Scleroderma
Hyderabad, India

My dear mother has been suffering from scleroderma for the past ten years. When I was a small boy, my mother's fingers would turn blue. This was more noticeable during winter when it was cold. She consulted all the specialists in the town where we were living, but none of the doctors diagnosed it as scleroderma or Raynaud's phenomenon.

In 1997, I secured a seat in a medical college in Hyderabad and enrolled for the MBBS degree course. I then took my mother to meet Dr. Narasimhalu in Rheumatology at Nizam Institute of Medical Sciences (NIMS) in Hyderabad. The doctor advised my mother to test for systemic lupus erythematosus (SLE). When we received the report, it showed the presence of SSA and SSB autoantibodies, and then my mother was diagnosed with scleroderma.

My mother's symptoms include Raynaud's phenomenon, digital infarcts, dyspnea (breathlessness) and slight fever. In one year, she has been treated for these symptoms and they are under control.

Many patients are undiagnosed or diagnosed very late. I am writing this story so that people will know that they have to approach the right specialist, as early as possible, and obtain the appropriate treatment.

Chapter 3

Systemic Scleroderma
Patient Stories

*I read your stories and hear your voices
and this, in itself, provides strength.*

— Jenny C. Besaw

Barbara "Bobbie" Thrasher
Missouri, USA

I was diagnosed with lupus in 1992. In November 1996, I was diagnosed with Raynaud's phenomenon, and my family doctor sent me to a rheumatology clinic.

My toes and fingers were so cold that they burned. There was an open sore on the end of my toe and one of my fingers. I was put on a blood thinner and soon after that, blood appeared in my stool. I became very weak and entered the hospital and was given many tests. They found that my stomach was weeping and I was given blood.

All this time, I began to notice my fingers were becoming curved and very sore. After six months, my finger and toe did heal with medication and prayer. By January 1998, I had full-blown scleroderma. I could not use my fingers to eat or write, nor did they have very much strength. They were very curved and stiff. I could stand, but I was put in a wheelchair to get around. My husband would push me because my fingers could not push the wheels.

I've been on an experimental medication for five months, and I have improved very much. I can type, write, and do many more things. I can walk a great distance. I have strength, and I have softened spots on my arms and legs. I do not need pain pills or "itch" pills.

I am not depressed. I live every day as if it is a blessing and, who knows, maybe a cure will be found. I will not give up. I love to hear my grandbabies call me, "Gammy." I have started collecting Beanie Babies. I may write a book about my childhood because I am blessed to use my fingers once again.

Update – September 1999

Now I am using my wheelchair only for very long walks. I can climb stairs, take my own bath, feed myself, comb my hair, and put in earrings. I no longer take pills for itching, nerves, or for the pain all over my body. I have gained strength in my arms and hands as well as the rest of my body. My fingers are still very curved and fit around a soda can, but nothing bigger. They are sore, but usable.

My doctor took me off the medication for six weeks to let my body rest. I now take only half a dose. This therapy has been very good for me. My doctor said we would give forty percent for the medicine and sixty percent for prayer. I am so happy with my progress that I wanted to give you all an update.

◆❖◆

Dawn Byron
Manitoba, Canada

I am a forty-nine-year-old woman recently diagnosed with early scleroderma. Although my problems with joint pain have been long-standing (approximately one and a half years), confirmation of my disease was made based on a positive scleroderma antibody found in my blood following testing for symptoms of Raynaud's phenomenon.

Since the onset of Raynaud's phenomenon in the fall of 2000, I have developed many symptoms associated with this disorder: swelling of the hands, long-standing pain in both shoulders (first thought to be a rotator cuff injury for which I am currently slated for arthroscopic surgery), bilateral knee and wrist pain, telangiectases, thickening of the skin on the hands, general muscle aches, weight loss, and fatigue.

I am fortunate that my general practitioner (GP) was familiar enough with my symptoms to draw the appropriate blood work, which ultimately led to my diagnosis by the rheumatologist to whom I was subsequently referred. Until further testing is completed, I am uncertain whether my disease is limited scleroderma or diffuse scleroderma.

As mentioned previously, I am currently awaiting surgery for what was thought to be a right rotator cuff injury. I now understand from my rheumatologist that this constant shoulder pain may, in fact, be a symptom of my disease. This, of course, raises the question, "Is surgery still an option?" Or do I forego such intervention, as it will not likely be of help?

Update – February 2002

It has been one year since my diagnosis was confirmed as diffuse scleroderma. The year can best be described as a rollercoaster ride of emotional uncertainty. However, during the course of that year, I have made a remarkable turnaround, both symptomatically and emotionally. Gone are the general muscle aches and pains, weight loss, and debilitating fatigue. I have regained eight of the almost eighteen pounds I had lost.

No doubt my medications have had a significant impact, but I know with complete certainty that the incredible emotional support of family and friends has been paramount in this improvement. Last March, I underwent the arthroscopic surgery of my left shoulder following lengthy discussion with both my rheumatologist and orthopedic surgeon. This surgery successfully corrected a rotator cuff injury totally unrelated to my scleroderma. I am now once more walking two to three miles a day and only miss a few miles during our coldest prairie winter days. Although my recent pulmonary function tests (PFTs) last month noted a slight deterioration in my lung capacity since last year's study, I am awaiting a CT scan to rule out alveolitis or pulmonary fibrosis.

I know stress can have debilitating effects on patients with autoimmune diseases. During this past year, I have dealt with my diagnosis of scleroderma, the death of a family member to cancer, life changes associated with the retirement of my husband, and the marriage of our only daughter. I truly believe that without a strong optimistic outlook and an I-cannot-let-this-defeat-me attitude, the improvement in my health would not have been possible. I know the road ahead is uncertain, but I plan to take each day, one at a time.

Flora Savini
Italy

I am a young woman, age twenty-three, and in August of 1999, I was admitted to Saint Anna Hospital in Ferrara and diagnosed with systemic sclerosis. I have also suffered from allergic asthma for around twenty years. At the moment, I have cyanosis of the hands with blue fingers and loss of strength. My breathing is currently under control. I must say, first of all, that before arriving at this diagnosis, I consulted many doctors at great expense and without satisfactory results.

I would like to understand much better the various aspects of my disease and the damage that it could cause me in order to answer my doubts, such as, "Will I be able to live a normal life?" I want to encourage all the people who suffer from scleroderma like me so that they manage to beat this disease.

Thank you for this space that was given to me to tell of my experiences and talk about my disease.

Giòvanna "Giò" Leonardo
Italy

I have been suffering from scleroderma since 1990. Currently, I take nifedipine, cortisone, aspirin, and calcium. For ten months of the year, I have infusions of Iloprost (prostacyclin) for three days per month, which I have to say has helped me a lot.

One needs to be steadfast and never lower one's guard. I thank all those people who help me to do my routine things every day.

Kathi Ragaglia
Oklahoma, USA

I am forty-three years old and have not felt well for ten years. I worked for the parks and recreation department in the city in which I lived for seventeen years, and that is where my story begins. I was a senior programs coordinator and also taught arts and crafts.

I started having problems with my hands not functioning. I was dropping things and had severe pain in my back. I was sent to a neurologist who did several tests and, at the time, he thought I had multiple sclerosis (MS) with severe carpal tunnel syndrome, bilaterally. MS was never confirmed.

I had bilateral surgery on my hands. A repeat EMG (a neuromuscular test) six months later found the condition was worse than before the surgery. There were other things going on: choking on everything I ate and a terrible burning sensation after eating. An MRI of the spine showed severe stenosis in almost every disc. An MRI of the brain showed nonspecific signal in the white matter, and an esophogram showed mild dysphagia (difficulty swallowing).

Then the send–you-to-all-the-specialists-we-can-think-of-because-we-just-do-not-know routine started. The family practice doctor said he felt it was fibromyalgia; the neurologist said probable MS; and the osteopath said, "I really think you have some connective tissue disease, but that is not my field and until you find out, I really do not suggest surgery on your back."

In the meantime, I had more tests. A pulmonary function test (PFT) showed a lung problem. Blood tests showed chronic hypoglycemia and a consistent low white blood cell count, along with a trace positive for cryoglobulin.

I felt like I was totally crazy and went to a psychologist, only to be told that depression is normal with these types of medical problems. I had to stop working because after eight hours, there was nothing left of me for my family. The fatigue is terrible, and I have had to learn how to pace myself, not easy with a Type A personality. Not knowing what is wrong is the worst feeling in the world. You know your body and you know something is wrong, but the professionals cannot seem to figure it out or agree on anything.

Finally, I got to see a rheumatologist who read my chart, which at this point was a novel, and he asked, "Have you ever heard of scleroderma?" My immediate response was, "You mean like that movie about Bob Saget's sister?" When he responded, "Yes," I was speechless.

I now understand not everyone with this disease has it quite the same way. It was such a relief to know what I was dealing with—that I am not crazy. At this point, I have never had positive antinuclear antibodies (ANA) or any of the antibody tests for scleroderma, but according my rheumatologist, just looking at my skin says all that needs to be said. I do have awful Raynaud's phenomenon, and telangiectases have started to appear all over my arms and face.

I have had several mammograms this year. My breasts on both sides are full of calcifications, which are not in the breast tissue, but not fully in the skin. My rheumatologist thinks it might be the scleroderma, and after a biopsy, the surgeon seems to agree. I know now that the brain MRI showed vascular attacks due to the scleroderma. The attacks result in terrible migraines. I have tried several antirheumatic drugs and so far nothing has worked. I have refused steroids, because after much research I decided the side effects of steroids were as bad as the disease.

I have agreed to try another arthritis medicine now, because my rheumatologist says we have got to slow this down. If it reduces the pain just one iota, it will be worth it.

Laura Witte
Nebraska, USA

I am fifty-three years old, a wife, mother, grandmother, and a real estate broker in Nebraska. I was recently diagnosed with scleroderma, perhaps diffuse scleroderma, as the pigmentation is symmetrical on both arms. I am glad to finally have an answer after years of tests with no results.

I am interested in knowing more about the first indications of bowel, heart, and lung involvement. I am presently on several antirheumatic medications, a sleep aid, and a drug to treat neuropathy (burning sensations.) For the last three years, I have had positive RH factors; they are now negative.

What has helped me most with the irritable bowel syndrome (IBS), believe it or not, is to have an instant breakfast shake every day.

I have a good attitude, a great husband, and a supportive and loving family. The hardest part of this was telling my family, as we knew someone who my age who recently passed away from complications of systemic scleroderma.

Pushpa Michael
Bangalore, India

It was the winter of 1982 when I first noticed my nails and fingers turning blue when exposed to the cold. I was twenty-one years old. The cold days in Calcutta are few—just a week or ten days a year—and the temperature does not go below fifteen to eighteen degrees Celsius (approximately sixty degrees Fahrenheit). I just ignored it. The next winter it happened again, but again I chose to ignore it.

A couple of months later in mid-1984, I noticed some white patches on my throat and at the back of my neck. It was uncanny because the patches seemed to be located exactly opposite each other! Thinking I had leukemia this time, I hit the panic button and visited my general practitioner. That is when I mentioned the blueness of my fingers during the last two winters.

After some inquiries, blood tests, and a skin biopsy, the end result was scleroderma with Raynaud's phenomenon. The doctor was very nice and asked if he could speak with my family. Sadly, my parents had passed away, and an older brother was too busy setting up his own family. The doctor spoke as gently as he could: I had been diagnosed with a rare, incurable illness for which little medication was known to help it. I inquired what caused it, but he said the cause is also unknown, thus, curing it was impossible. I did not tell anyone about my diagnosis as I was not sure, nor did I understand the seriousness of the illness.

I was given many medicines, and told not to touch or try to hold anything cold. One medicine gave me terrible heart palpitations, and it seemed as if my eardrums would burst, so I asked to stop it. But clever me, without telling the doctor, I stopped all allopathic medicines and tried homeopathy because I was more worried about the white patches than blue fingers!

I had worked as a telephone-cum-telex operator for over nine years, the latter part of which was in an air-conditioned room. My fingers started to swell and become painful. Typing was difficult as a couple of fingers began to bend inward. My friends and colleagues began to notice and asked me about it. I explained my illness the best way I could, but realized I was not getting it across to them.

Meanwhile, the white patches disappeared, never to reappear. All this time I was still on homeopathy.

During the late 1980s, some wonderful things happened, and I had a proposal from a believer. Before accepting, I told him about my illness and gave him time to think things over. He said something so touching and lovely then: "We cannot foresee our future, but we can accept our present and let God take control of the rest."

We were married in October 1990 and moved to Bangalore, India. Now in a new state, I needed a new doctor for consultation. I ended up in St. John's Hospital where I underwent some blood tests, an endoscopy, ECG, and another skin biopsy. The result was that the scleroderma and Raynaud's phenomenon had spread far and wide. I was advised to take some medication again, but would not. Steroids were also offered on a trial basis, but I refused.

Then we got the good news that I was expecting a baby. I was told to abort the baby because giving birth would have a serious effect on my illness. All the same, as long as the baby was okay, I was willing to take the risk. So with the help of my gynecologist came our pride and joy on Christmas Eve 1991 by Cesarean section.

When our baby girl was just three months old, my husband changed jobs. It did not work out and he was out of work for a year, during which worry and anxiety took a severe toll on my health. Over the next two years, I lost weight dramatically and was just a bag of bones! Until our baby was over three years old, I did everything for her, as well as the cooking, etc. Soon after that, my ankles started swelling and became so painful I could hardly walk; thus began the shuffling.

Now, almost twenty years since my illness was diagnosed, my condition is like this: I can open my mouth less than two fingers (vertically) wide, I can barely turn my head from side to side, and my shoulders are beginning to get stiff. My elbows are at an angle and I cannot straighten my arms, even if one tries to pull them straight. My wrists do not flex at all. My left hand is closed like a fist; my right hand is partially closed like a claw. Thankfully, my back is straight and my hip joints are okay. My knees and ankles are swollen and painful, and my toes are crooked and bent.

As for medication, I only take ibuprofen, which has increased from one to four tablets a day over the years. I took no other medication from the time I was expecting to the date of this writing. For extreme pain, I apply ointment and keep the area bandaged until I return to my usual painful self.

The good part is that my internal organs are okay, the scleroderma has stabilized, and I can still type with the help of two chopsticks. I can proudly say that I have written this story myself.

Better still is my family. Piers, my husband, says he loves me more now (his very words) than when we met and married for the way I manage and cope daily. He helps out with chores before he goes to his office. Persis, our daughter who has never seen me well, helps in any way she can when she returns from school. During the daytime, the maid comes to do the other work and the cooking, leaving me with very little to do.

But the best part is that I believe in miracles and know I will be healed soon. My message is: Have faith. Be strong! Do not give up!

Valeria Macali
Italy

I am a twenty-one-year-old woman and at the age of nine, I was diagnosed with systemic sclerosis. From then I have been treated at the A. Gemelli Hospital in Rome. I need to be admitted once or twice per year to have all the routine tests and undergo various treatments, including medications and various creams.

At the moment, my situation is as follows: loss of the elasticity of the skin of my face, hands and forearms; reduced esophageal motility; gastroesophageal reflux; chronic gastritis; and greatly impaired circulation in my fingers and toes.

In April 1999, I started treatment with intravenous vasodilators at intervals of three months, so for every two months that I am at home, I spend about a month in the hospital. I do not want to try to explain how much this disease has cost me in terms of physical and psychological suffering and I cannot find suitable words to describe how it has altered my life.

I would like to find out about all the possible treatments for this disease, all the centers that are interested in it (in Italy and abroad) as well as all the tests necessary to ascertain the damage the disease could cause. I would also like to know if any center exists (perhaps not too far from Rome) where I could get adequate physiotherapy for my face and hands, given that I even find it tiring to roll up spaghetti and I cannot even manage to laugh because I get immediate cramps in my cheeks.

I would also like to say that my friends have played a fundamental role on this journey of mine in that they have never allowed me to feel alone for even a moment. Without their presence and support, I would never have been able to overcome the humiliation and suffering of my recent admissions to hospital.

To all the people with my disease, I would like to say one thing: Don't let scleroderma wear out your heart as it does your body. A sincere thanks to all of you for the help that you are giving me.

◆❖◆

Carol Langenfeld
Ohio, USA

Carol Langenfeld is co-author of the book entitled, Living Better: Every Patient's Guide to Living with Illness.

People tell me I have earned my credentials as a "certified patient" the hard way after almost twenty-five years. Many times I have wished I could drop my diseased body off at the laundry and pick it up the next day, fresh and clean and ready to face the world anew.

The birth of my son, Eric, in 1979 was a joyful occasion; an experience to celebrate and feel grateful. Six weeks after his birth, I could hardly pick him up. My hands were painful, hot, and so swollen I could not shut them. I frequently opened and closed my hands to try to relax the stiffness, hoping the pain would ease so I could safely pick him up, unpin his diaper, change him, and feed him. The winter of 1979-1980 was the winter of the energy crisis, and my hands were constantly blue due to the government's request to keep thermostats as low as fifty-five degrees at night!

Diagnosis was not easy. The test results did not fit into a diagnosis; I looked fine on paper! It was hard for my family to understand why I complained so much when the tests showed nothing was wrong. Eventually, my family doctor called my condition rheumatoid arthritis. I knew that did not really fit my symptoms. His treatments were not very helpful and I continued to get worse.

Friends and family urged me to go to a specialist. I resisted, but eventually, a year later, agreed to see a rheumatologist. This doctor looked at me and immediately recognized that I had a connective tissue disease called scleroderma. I had seen it described in an Arthritis Foundation's brochure, but had no idea the impact the diagnosis would have on my life. Very few people are aware of this disease now and even fewer knew of it in 1979. I often tell friends that scleroderma is a cousin of lupus, because people are much more likely to have heard of lupus.

This life-changing illness hit me in the first several years of my son's life. I was young, in my early and middle twenties. Though doctors and researchers may have more specific explanations and understandings about this disease, what I knew at the time was that I desperately hurt. I was always cold. My hands were blue, and I had ulcers on the tips of my fingers.

I had terrible acid indigestion. Swallowing was painful. Breathing deeply made my chest ache.

In addition, I began to frequently feel strange palpitations in my chest. Eventually, I blacked out at home, and my family called the emergency squad to take me to the emergency room. Six weeks later, after confirming that my heart did not reliably conduct the electrical impulse to cause my heart to beat, I had surgery to implant a cardiac pacemaker. That was the beginning of some life-threatening events that still happen occasionally. I am absolutely dependent on my pacemaker: if it does not beat, my heart does not beat.

Today, I still have diffuse scleroderma (although it is not progressing) and its residual damage. Now more than twenty years later, I still have aches and pains, tire easily and take naps, and require visits to six or seven specialists. I take twelve different prescriptions, give or take a few depending on the day, and I still take a nap on most days. Most of my organ systems have been affected, including heart, lungs, gastrointestinal tract (including Barrett's esophagus), endocrine disorders (thyroiditis and early menopause), Sjögren's, Raynaud's phenomenon, depression, and some skin involvement.

With the help and encouragement of friends and family, I have been a mother for twenty-four years and a wife for twenty-seven years. I completed my Master's degree in counseling in 1996 and now work at my church counseling on a very part-time basis.

With a lot of help from my friends, I made a choice along with my husband and son to find opportunity hidden within the crisis of my illness. We found friends, family, and faith that we may not have discovered had scleroderma not happened. We found inner strength and capabilities we could not have imagined. I certainly never expected to write a book! Along with my husband, who suffers from a pituitary tumor and complicating endocrine disorders, I have written *Living Better: Every Patient's Guide to Living with Illness*.

Scleroderma is life changing! I encourage each of my fellow scleroderma friends to take one day at a time, learn as much as you can about your illness, seek the best medical care you can, and take the best possible care of yourself each and every day.

◆ ❖ ◆

Deborah Peck
Tennessee, USA

I first noticed my hands turning white after my father's funeral in 1992. Of course, all my expert friends attributed the color change to stress.

In the fall of 1998, my hands began to turn blue when exposed to cold. A rheumatologist diagnosed me with primary Raynaud's phenomenon. In March 2000, one fingertip turned blue and stayed blue with a decrease in temperature for about two weeks. I saw a rheumatologist who ran lots of tests, just to be safe, even though he believed I was only suffering from primary Raynaud's phenomenon.

We were surprised that I tested positive for SCL-70, which is a scleroderma antibody. The rheumatologist said I have a chance of developing systemic sclerosis later in life. I did research and began to share symptoms with my rheumatologist I thought might be relevant.

I have noticed in the last year or so that I occasionally have audible gasps for air. My finger is still not well after three months. The rheumatologist ordered a chest X ray. It was suspicious, and the PFT was not normal.

I have an appointment with the rheumatologist in August 2000. What should I expect? What should I ask? What tests need to be performed?

In June of 2000, my patient story was posted on the website. At some point, I questioned what it meant to have a positive SCL-70.

Shelley Ensz sent me a warm, loving, and caring response and for that, I would like to thank her. She quoted text by two physicians on scleroderma and, of course, advised me to talk with my doctor.

I promptly called him and gave him the information she had given me. I told him I had been experiencing shortness of breath for a year. He said if it would make me feel any better, he would order a chest X ray. I said it would make me feel better. The chest X ray was suspicious; the PFT was not normal; and the high-resolution CT scan showed inflammation in my lungs.

Thanks to this, I received a quick diagnosis of diffuse systemic sclerosis with lung involvement in August 2000. I began a series of six low-dose chemotherapy treatments four weeks ago. Upon completion, I will have another CT scan to determine what difference the chemotherapy has made.

My rheumatologist is following the NIH criteria for treatment based upon the success lupus patients have experienced with this protocol. I am also searching for alternative medicine and looking into natural healing.

Thanks a million for your help and your website!

Update – February 2002

I had another PFT one year ago after the six chemotherapy treatments. It showed there had been no change. I had two more low-dose treatments and then moved from Germany back to America in June 2001.

I finally saw a rheumatologist in December 2001. She recommended that I see a pulmonologist, which I did in January 2002. I had another PFT, which showed no progression of my condition since August 2000. Hooray!

I had a bronchoscopy and a lung biopsy to confirm my diagnosis, and it was positive for scleroderma-induced alveolitis. The pulmonologist and rheumatologist both suggested I take steroids for two months and have another PFT. I refused to take the steroids. I have learned that studies show that steroids are not good for people with my condition.

I regularly pray for healing and attend church. I am a member of the local YMCA and I exercise. I am taking a lot of vitamins and minerals, and I refer often to books on integrative medicine. I just ordered a breathing CD, and I have begun to take a Chinese herbal blend for healthy lungs.

I try to live one day at a time and trust God to heal me, which may be with chemotherapy and/or a combination of other treatments. So as my personal pathway to healing is revealed, I intend to follow it.

Update – February 2002

I just received a call this week from my rheumatologist in Nashville. She contacted Dr. Barbara White in Maryland, who thinks I have not received enough chemotherapy, so I will begin this week taking it daily for eighteen months.

There is a clinical trial going on at Virginia Hospital in Nashville by Drs. King and Strickland. A woman with whom I have spoken said she looked like a burn victim and that within a matter of weeks, this procedure helped her return to virtual normalcy. I will call my doctor again and ask about this treatment for scleroderma-induced lung disease.

I have some skin tightening, but at forty-four years of age, it is flattering at this point. Perhaps the cosmetic and pharmaceutical giants are aware of this, and they are pouring research dollars into finding a cure, which will lead to bottling and selling what induces this process in the first place!

◆ ❖ ◆

Gregory Ferrata
Diffuse Scleroderma, Lung Transplant Patient
Texas, USA

I was diagnosed with diffuse scleroderma in October of 1997. I am now forty-one years old, and married with four wonderful children.

I was always in great shape. I was a scholarship linebacker for the University of Texas back in the Earl Campbell days. Since then, I have taken a great deal of pride in my physical shape and abilities. I was very in tune with my body.

In July of 1997, I enrolled in a martial arts class. I felt I was losing some flexibility, and I thought the stretching would help. Little did I know the tightness and loss in my range of motion was due to scleroderma, not just age. My next symptom was shortness of breath.

I was lucky in that I was properly diagnosed quickly. Lung X rays showed fibrosis, and pulmonary function tests (PFTs) showed a severe reduction in lung capacity and oxygen diffusion.

Things started to go downhill from there. In May of 2000, my doctor informed me that my condition was severe, and that a lung transplant might be my only option for survival. I was not ready to deal with that. I considered the options and asked Dr. Frank C. Arnett to make the necessary arrangements to see if I was a candidate for a transplant.

I was evaluated by a great team of transplant specialists at Methodist Hospital in Houston and was approved for the operation. The call came just fifteen days after I was listed on the transplant network. What a miracle! July 25, 2000, is a day I will never forget. I was eating dinner at 6:30 and on the operating table by 8:30. My new lung was in San Antonio; I was in Houston. I prayed and they put me under. I awoke and was sore as heck, but I could feel the new lung working! I stayed in the hospital for twenty-eight days, and I am pleased to say, I am making excellent progress.

I have to take a lot of drugs, but I can ride my bike and take walks with my family. I am truly blessed. Scleroderma has not attacked my new lung, and I am hopeful that it will remain unaffected. My heartfelt thanks go out to all the doctors and staff members who have helped put my life back together.

I have been told that transplants are not very common for scleroderma patients, but consult your doctor concerning this matter. I do not know how long my new lease on life will last, but I do know that we are making progress toward solving the mystery of scleroderma.

Make the most of every day. Each day is a chance to do something for which you can be proud. Keep up the good fight!

Hiwee Be-Maria
Amman, Jordan

I am Iraqi and about sixteen years ago, I began my struggle with scleroderma. I had very good doctors in Iraq. They told me what would happen to me in the future. Unfortunately, the bad circumstances in my country prevented our doctors from getting the latest medicines that could help to improve my status. So I came to Amman, Jordan in 1991 with my sister, Suzan, with the hope of getting a visa to any other country in which I could be treated, at least to minimize the amount of the pain I feel every minute of my life.

In my first years in Amman, I saw some doctors, but my health got worse with the medications they gave me, so I stopped taking them. Besides, the medicine also cost too much.

Now my whole body, especially my hands, has become hard like stone. I cannot eat anything, but soup. Even with soup, I have acid in my stomach, especially at night. My face has changed and I have lost a lot of weight.

I know there is no treatment for this disease, and I know also I will never return back as I was before, unless by a miracle. All I want is to stop my pain.

For all the people with illnesses in this world, I am praying to get rid of their pain. I have hope that my Lord will listen to my crying and that He may do something to ease my pain.

Marilyn Jack
Ontario, Canada

When I was diagnosed with diffuse scleroderma two and a half years ago, it was no surprise at all. I had known for several years something was wrong—I just could not convince anyone else of it, until one day at work, when my coworkers noticed that while sitting having coffee, I was very short of breath.

As a nurse, you would think I would have picked up on this myself. At the time, I also had a very sore back and could not remember injuring it. I was sent off the ward and instructed to have blood work done to find out what was going on.

At this point, I had severe heartburn, shortness of breath, severe diarrhea, and many little things going on. My blood showed a positive ANA titre. From there I had several other tests done: bone scan; MRI of the head, neck, and stomach; CAT scan. You name it, and I had it done.

When everything came back, I was told I had scleroderma, the bad kind. My heart, lungs, and kidneys were involved. I had reflux and managed to aspirate, which put me back in the hospital once again.

At this time, I was told there was not much they could do for me. I was forty-one years old and that was probably as far as I was going. I took this lightly and was not going to lie back and die.

I fought them the whole way. I started having trouble with my breathing; every time I laid down, I would lose my breath. It felt as if a flap was closing over and I had a very difficult time getting my breath back.

I was sent to a sleep disorders doctor, who discovered I have severe sleep apnea, which could not be controlled with a continuous positive airway pressure (CPAP) monitor. I had a tracheostomy because the damage that was being done was irreversible and causing brain damage.

Since my tracheostomy, I feel like a new person. My skin has softened somewhat. I still have reflux, but not as severe. I feel like I have recaptured ten years. I have stuck faithfully to the medication the doctors have prescribed.

Things are looking up right now! Presently, I have six doctors looking after me: a rheumatologist, respirologist, gastroenterologist, sleep disorders doctor, trachea surgeon, and a gynecologist, along with my family doctor. They all stay in touch with each other and discuss any changes made as a team.

Things are great again. I can even remember things that happened last week, last month, and even some things that happened last year. I have been doing a lot of searching on the Internet trying to find more information on this and I am finding this website very informative.

Update – December 2000

Recently, I agreed to take an antidepressant medication and things are even better than they were before. Finally, I am able to get some weight off and I can see a real difference.

My skin is not tight and bound down as it was. It is actually becoming movable, more pliable! My stomach problems continue to bother me, but they are under control with medication. I have not aspirated in months. This is unbelievable.

I continue to feel better since my tracheostomy. It seems to be doing its job. I am breathing much easier and able to sleep at night, something I have not done for years.

All in all, the improvements are outstanding! I would really like to talk with people who have scleroderma, but particularly those who have diffuse scleroderma.

I am from Canada and I have been working with the Arthritis Society trying to find a support group, but our very large town does not offer much.

Update – January 2002

A lot has happened since I last updated this story. I continue to have problems with aspirating. In September 2001, I had a G-J (gastrostomyjeju-nostomy) tube inserted into my stomach. This was done because the motility in my stomach is poor and foods were not digesting. I was having difficulty with swallowing, choking, and aspirating on everything.

I had my throat stretched several times, yet I continued to choke. Since I have had the tube, my stomach feels much better. I am not having as much discomfort and things are looking better once again.

I still have the tracheostomy. I was hoping this would only be temporary, but I guess I was wrong about that. I am still having problems with shortness of breath. Right now, my biggest problem is water retention. But I should not really complain about it, because I feel too good to complain. Take care and do not give up the fight. There is always a brighter tomorrow, if you want it!

◆ ❖ ◆

Rosellen Hartman
Ohio, USA

I was diagnosed with scleroderma in January of 1994. I was thirty-two years old at the time. My symptoms started when I was cold or stressed. My hands would turn purple, almost black. I also had a wound on the top of my index finger on my left hand that would not heal, and it was very painful.

I went to the doctor then not only because of my hands, but because I had a cold that I was nursing for three months. I was getting frequent nosebleeds that were pretty intense. My family doctor did some blood tests and found my ANA and sedimentation rates were elevated. He suspected scleroderma.

He referred me to a doctor I had seen fifteen years prior, a rheumatologist who treated scleroderma patients, or so he said. When I was sixteen years old, I had surgery to remove an ovarian cyst the size of a basketball weighing in at eighteen pounds. It was after this surgery that I developed swollen hands that ached constantly. This progressed to all the joints in my body, and this rheumatologist said, "If you do not lose the weight, it will be like hell on roller skates." He ignored the fact I had elevated tests even at that point.

He was not able to help me this time, either. I was very scared, as my hands were getting worse. I was having a hard time breathing, and I felt miserable all the time. Then I located my current doctor, a rheumatologist who specializes in and conducts research in scleroderma right in my city. A godsend! He has helped me more than I can say, not only through his obvious knowledge of the disease, but with his compassion and humanitarian qualities!

He has treated me successfully for the lung involvement. I was put on chemotherapy for two years and my pulmonary function tests (PFTs) are back in the normal range. My situation includes vascular involvement, and I have fought ulcers on my fingers throughout the entire illness. My first severe ulcer finally healed after a year. I was not so lucky with the next ulcer. It had advanced such that the nail fell off, and the first third of my finger was covered with a mere sheath of skin that was black and becoming gangrenous.

I was working at the time as a veterinary technician for a busy emergency clinic with animals that really did not care if it really hurt when they smashed your hand against the treatment tables. After trying for a year and a half to get the finger to heal, the decision was made to amputate. The pain that kept me up in tears all night, every night, was finally gone. Yes, it took some time to get used to the finger being gone, but let's face it, the finger was never going to be the same anyway.

I have had other trials and tribulations that have lead me to conclude that working like I was accustomed, was no longer possible. I have filed for disability. I keep busy with other activities, including working out at the spa four or five times a week. I have found some time for me now and with the Lord's help, my life is heading in a new direction. I will accept what comes and learn to live with it as we all do. I wish all of you the best.

Aileen Hickey
NSW, Australia

I was fifty-three years old in January 2002. I have a delightful husband, two daughters, and four grandchildren, with a fifth on the way. Scleroderma has been a bit of a bumpy path for me, but I think I am now at peace with my monster. I suppose my story begins when I was a small child.

We lived in a place with cold, wet, and frosty winters. They were miserable for me. I always had such cold hands and feet, which were covered in chilblains.

It was not until I was about thirty that other symptoms started to occur. I was diagnosed with acid reflux and told to take antacids—everything would be fine.

I always had aching joints, and I would hate to count the number of X rays that were taken looking for arthritis that was never there. I just gave up going to the doctor in the end and put up with it all, until my hands decided they would give up being useful and turned into numb lumps at the end of my arms. I had to go to the doctor then. He took one look at them and said it was Raynaud's phenomenon. He would do some blood tests as sometimes lupus accompanies Raynaud's phenomenon. I had heard of lupus, but did not know much about it.

I was very nervous when I called for the blood test results. What a troubling conversation that was. He told me the tests showed positive ANA. He then proceeded to say, "I really do not know what to do with you. Maybe you had better make an appointment, and we will see who we can send you to." As you can probably imagine, I was rather puzzled and anxious over all this. I went to see him and was referred to another doctor. He told me I did not have lupus; I had CREST.

He explained that it was like a cousin to lupus. He talked a bit about T cells, which went straight over my head. He gave me some tablets that he said would help the Raynaud's phenomenon and, if I had any problems, to go back to my general practitioner (GP). At no time was the word scleroderma mentioned. I assumed all I had to worry about was Raynaud's phenomenon.

The tablets did not help, so I went back to my GP. I tried numerous different medications with no result. I was then sent for Guanethidine blocks, of which I had three, also with no result. At the same time, the pain in my joints was getting worse. I spoke to my GP about it, and he seemed to think it was the work I was doing. He gave me anti-inflammatories. Wow! My stomach did not love those. At no time was I told that painful joints were part of my disease.

My husband and I both worked very long hours at fairly stressful jobs. We had our own small, stone fruit property that we were slowly building up, and we also worked away from our farm. He worked in a bowling club, and I worked ten hours a day, six days a week as a packing manager for a large grape and avocado export property.

I was always exhausted and in a lot of pain. I handled the pain by working harder until the pain turned to a warm fluid in my body. That was okay until I stopped, then it was agonizing. I could not sleep because the pressure of my own body on the bed hurt too much, so I was existing on four to five hours of sleep a night.

Then, it all came tumbling down. Fatigue hit in a big way and I could not eat; I always felt full. I lost eight kilograms in six weeks. I went back to the GP only to hear him ask if I was worried about something. Worry can make you tired and lose your appetite. I left his office feeling let down.

I gave up work thinking I would get better, but the fatigue continued and so did the lack of appetite. Then, a boon happened when we got connected to the Internet. I typed in the search term 'CREST' and sat in front of my computer in a state of shock. This was the first time I realized I had scleroderma and what that meant to my life. Thankfully, my husband was not home, so I had time to cry it out, sit and look at what may be in store for me, and then compose myself. I printed out some of the basic information and made an appointment to see my GP. When presented with the information, he asked if he could keep it. He said he really did not know very much about scleroderma and it made for interesting reading.

This man had been treating me for five years, but knew nothing! I felt angry, sick, and betrayed. How could he keep me as his patient under these circumstances? Why did he not refer me to a specialist? Perhaps he really did not know how serious scleroderma could be. He may even have been as ignorant as me and thought the Raynaud's phenomenon was the only symptom that came with it.

My husband and I had to make a decision about our future. I could no longer work on our property, and the extreme weather was physically hard on me. With many tears, we decided to sell our beautiful property and move closer to our daughters and grandchildren.

I was very lucky to find a GP who immediately sent me to a specialist. Oh, it is a wonderful feeling to have a doctor tell me that I was not imagining things; that everything I was experiencing was because of scleroderma! He monitors me closely with a range of blood tests every three months, a yearly pulmonary function test (PFT), and an echocardiogram. I am treated so well and bless my luck in finding him.

The fatigue is terrible and never lets up. It has changed my whole life and the way I do things. We never plan anything ahead, but take things day by day. I went through a period of terrible grieving, then anger at losing my mobility. I have always been a doer, always on the move. I loved bush walking, swimming, all outdoor activities and, in one fell swoop, it had all been taken away. I was left a spectator.

I have come to terms with it now and take great pleasure in the slower things in life, like bird watching, my frog pond, and my computer.

My stomach is a major problem, as it does not empty. I am on medications for it, but it is no better. I am thin and will just have to stay that way. At mealtimes, I have no appetite and must force myself to eat. To no avail, my gastroenterologist sent me to a dietitian with the hope he could sort out a food regimen to help put on some weight.

One great bonus to come out of all this is the friends I have made around the world. During a very low ebb, I found a website and submitted my story. I was overwhelmed by the response, and I now have a wonderful circle of people to whom I write regularly. I also started my own website, Scleroderma and You, as therapy for myself and, after a very slow beginning, it has grown rapidly.

It has taken me a long time to stop fighting against scleroderma and to start accepting the way I now must live my life. I willingly let my family help me instead of trying to do it all myself. My daughter told me she used to go home and cry because she felt so helpless watching me try to do things for myself and I would get cranky when she would try to help. I think it is very important for our families to be a part of our illness and not shut them out. They hurt, too.

Each day brings new challenges with our disease, but as long as we face them with a positive attitude and a smile, we will overcome all obstacles.

◆ ❖ ◆

Angiola Sbolli
Italy

I was diagnosed with progressive systemic sclerosis in 1997, when I was fifty-seven. The diagnosis was made at the first visit as the disease was already in an advanced state, and the signs of it were very evident.

The symptoms, that I had ignored for so long, had already been present for many years: thickening of the skin on my abdomen, swelling and pain in my hands with stiffness and ulceration, persistent cough, and general fatigue. After an acute phase, today (April 2000) it seems that the disease has stabilized for the moment, but the damage has not cleared up. I suffer from marked lung fibrosis, which forces me to use oxygen continuously. I also have reflux esophagitis, mild cardiac involvement, serious visceral involvement and widespread pain.

I take both steroids and vasodilator therapy with nifedipine, which has greatly improved the Raynaud's phenomenon in my hands.

This is my story. I would very much like to find other people who find themselves in a similar situation, so that we can take a load off one another's minds.

◆ ❖ ◆

Arianna Balduino
Italy

My name is Arianna and I am a twenty-six-year-old woman. In September 2000, I was finally diagnosed with a form of progressive systemic sclerosis, but everything had started a good three years earlier with the sudden whitening of a finger while I was walking along the street downtown with my university friends.

When I told my family doctor about this strange phenomenon, he replied that I should wear gloves because it was cold outside! After a few months, other fingers became affected by this phenomenon, this time associated with pain. Nothing! No one could tell me what it was!

Suddenly in April 2000, I started to feel generally stiff. I couldn't bend over to carry out the usual domestic tasks, my ankles were always swollen and my hands began to deform and swell. My mother noticed a certain change in my face, as my nose got thinner and my mouth became tighter.

I got to the point where I couldn't get up from a chair without grabbing hold of something to pull myself up. I felt humiliated! How was it possible that a girl of twenty-four could have the energy of an eighty year old?

Without sending me for tests, my doctor told me that maybe I had rheumatoid arthritis. Everything changed after I met my current rheumatologist, who understood the cause of my suffering by simply looking at my face. Now I take so many medicines that I cannot keep count of them, and I have physiotherapy. I have met some wonderful people (the doctors at the hospital, the nurses and the physiotherapists, and the patients at the day hospital).

Unfortunately, all this is still not enough, as the disease is not going into remission. On the contrary, it is progressing inexorably.

Last month, my rheumatologist told me that I have an inflammation of the lungs, and that if I do not want to end up on oxygen therapy, I have to start a new treatment that can have serious side effects on my ovaries. The world fell down on me. I had still hoped to live a normal life, marry and have children!

Maybe I was a bit presumptuous, but thinking about everything again now, what I want is to struggle against this disease to stop it from beating me. I love you all!

◆ ❖ ◆

Awilda E. Berríos Burgos
CREST and Morphea Scleroderma
Puerto Rico

I am fifty-three years old. In 1971, I had the first symptoms of Raynaud's phenomenon. I was young, single, and starting my first job as an accountant at a university. I noticed that when I held objects, such as the phone, or when the weather was cold, or when I was in an air-conditioned room, my fingers would turn white or deep blue (almost purple). For that reason, I went to the doctor, and he said this was a symptom of Raynaud's phenomenon. He also said I did not have the illness, just the symptoms.

In 1973, I developed an esophageal hernia with reflux and stomach pain. Doctors said I also had many stomach ulcers. Medications controlled these symptoms, and I continued to live my life normally.

I was a smoker for twenty-five years, and my condition grew worse. In 1988, I had a black heart-finger (middle finger) that stayed that way for a week. I tried many alternative medicines trying to heal this condition, even acupuncture. Finally a doctor took me to the surgery room and injected a liquid in my neck to help increase my blood circulation. It was a very bad, painful, and dangerous solution. It was supposed to be done three times, but luckily by the second injection, my finger had returned to normal. This procedure scared me so much that since that day, I never smoked again. I continued a normal life with Raynaud's phenomenon episodes, reflux, and ulcers.

In 1997, when Hurricane Hortense struck our island, I had double pneumonia. The day after the storm I was rushed to the emergency room and hospitalized. I was very ill. In the hospital I was diagnosed with CREST and then with scleroderma.

I was out of work for about four months. It was not easy for me because I had always been a hard worker. I worked in high positions—finance director, system and procedures director, budget director—which included many stressful duties. I had to change many things in the way I did my job in order to continue working.

Since then I have developed morphea, cellulite, and phlebitis in my legs. At times my legs are red with other painful, dark marks. The marks start small and then grow. Eventually, the skin becomes hard as a rock.

I developed rosacea on my face, so I am always watching my skin. I also have developed little finger ulcers. Asthma is another illness for which I have been hospitalized many times. My body is always cold, including my toes. Sometimes I woke up very tired, but still had to go to work. I tried to do my best in my job and thankfully, I managed to complete my thirty years in public service work. I retired from service on December 31, 2001. I did not want to stop working, but it was the best thing for me. Now I feel free of stressful situations.

I have ups and downs, but by reading others' testimonies, I am not so bad off. I try to feel fine and keep going. When I can dance, I dance. When I feel tired, I simply do nothing. No matter what, I do my best.

I am now working as an independent travel agent from my home. Without much investment, I am doing what I always wanted to do and I love it! I just want to keep working since I enjoy being useful. I am planning to go on vacation soon, thanks to this job. I recommend a home-based business. It works for me and has been a new, lifetime opportunity.

I think I have been blessed because, after all, I have accomplished my duties as wife, mother, and public servant. I am still here enjoying the beauty of life. And no matter how I feel, I keep on! May God bless all of you!

Barbara Lowe
England

I suppose I always knew something was wrong. To my friends, I seemed to be a hypochondriac because every day it seemed like there was something new.

I was nineteen when I first noticed my fingers turning white. I now recognize that these were classic Raynaud's phenomenon attacks. I always felt so tired, and I seemed to suffer colds much worse than anyone else. I felt permanently run down.

It was not until I married and became pregnant that I started to experience real problems. I was healthy all through the pregnancy, but soon after giving birth, my health just seemed to go downhill.

In 1995, I had a serious bout of pneumonia that never really improved. It led to asthma and breathing problems. I also had problems with my esophagus and found that eating became increasingly more difficult.

A doctor once said to me, "I think you may have scleroderma," but it was not mentioned again. I suffered another bout of pneumonia in 1997, and again it took time to recover. The word scleroderma was mentioned yet again, and I even wrote the word down because I could not remember it.

In 1999, my symptoms became worse. I asked the consultant who was treating my swallowing problems what he thought was causing the symptoms. It was then he finally referred me to a rheumatologist.

A simple blood test clearly showed the antibodies responsible for scleroderma. It was the year 2000; diagnosis had taken more than twenty years.

I know I am lucky because I have limited involvement. But that does not mean the pain is any less. I cannot do the things I know I should be able to do. My eating has gotten worse, and I can only tolerate liquefied food. My weight has dropped considerably in the last year, three stones, in fact. My Raynaud's phenomenon is worsening and requires hospital treatment, especially in the winter.

I am always interested in other people's stories and journeys to diagnosis. I have a very supportive family in my husband and eleven-year-old daughter. I have everything to live for, and I am going to live it the best I can.

◆❖◆

Brenda C. Stamper
Ohio, USA

I was diagnosed with limited scleroderma, Raynaud's phenomenon, and CREST syndrome on October 2, 2001. I am fifty-six years old, married with two grown children (a boy and a girl), and a grandson.

At this point, what I know about this disease is what I have found on this website. This is a wonderful site for people. I feel much better mentally for being in the know.

I have been sick for five or six years, telling doctors how much pain I have and that my fingers are sensitive to cold. I went to three doctors in six years and finally I was referred to a specialist.

I am new to this so I do not have a lot of information to contribute. At this time, my doctor has me on medication for the Raynaud's, and has warned me to stay warm at all times.

Update – November 2001

I went back to the doctor in October and was told I also have fibromyalgia. I have irritable bowel syndrome (IBS), sleep apnea, thyroid problems, and diabetes. Maybe this information will help with statistics. It seems lots of people have IBS and sleep apnea before symptoms of scleroderma.

I am reading some things online that are frightening. What am I to expect?

◆ ❖ ◆

Carol Curtin
Melbourne, Australia

For as long as I can remember, I always felt cold. I was the child at school who sat at the back of the class, not because I was inattentive, but because that was often closest to the old hot water panel that warmed the classroom.

By the time I was thirteen, I was hiding my stiff, white, and painful hands in gloves and in pockets. Shortly after this, I developed the same symptoms in my feet and at times, walking became difficult and painful.

At nineteen, I was on all sorts of medication to relieve symptoms of what was finally diagnosed as Raynaud's phenomenon. My feet suffered so badly that I underwent a chemical sympathectomy to alleviate the pain and problems with walking. This was successful in the short term. Thankfully, the Raynaud's phenomenon in my feet has gradually improved over the years.

In 1992, at age thirty, I gave birth to my second child, Max. With Raynaud's phenomenon still a problem, I was undergoing a treatment that required a drug to be intravenously fed into each hand over a period of weeks. This treatment was supposed to keep the Raynaud's phenomenon attacks at bay during the cold months.

It was during one of these treatments that a very young and observant doctor noticed the red spots (telangiectases) on my hands and the contraction of a finger. The Raynaud's phenomenon, with all its problems, soon took a backseat as a rheumatologist told me that blood tests revealed that I had, in fact, a very rare disease called scleroderma.

Thinking she would follow with something like, "And if you take these tablets, those unsightly spots will go away, no big deal really." I was unprepared for what actually followed when she said, "It is an incurable disease that little is known about with an uncertain future, given the possible directions the disease could take." Tests followed and, finally it was revealed that for me, the prognosis was good. I had the CREST variant.

It is now ten years since I was diagnosed and while I present every one of C, R, E, S, and T of CREST, I am managing the disease. I have taken medication since my diagnosis and this has worked well. I have problems with gastroesophageal reflux, but antacids and diet modification keep that under control.

My Raynaud's phenomenon is still a bother, and the tight, glossy skin does nothing to enhance the beauty of my corpse-like hands. My daughter, who is fifteen, and my son, who is nine, always hold my hands when we are out—partly because they love me, but more because they know that they can use their body heat to keep an attack at bay for me.

The only problem I have developed recently has been debilitating migraines that a neurologist suspects may be triggered like Raynaud's phenomenon, by temperature change. A migraine attack will present all the signs of a stroke including memory loss, visual disturbance, loss of speech, loss of feeling down one side, and, of course, the pain that follows.

I have worked full time as a senior secondary school teacher since I was twenty (I am now forty). I have only taken short breaks to have my children. Scleroderma and Raynaud's phenomenon have not robbed me of a fulfilling career. Over the years, my students have been astonished by my hands, particularly during a Raynaud's phenomenon attack when I cannot hold a piece of chalk to write on the board or a pen to mark the roll.

Necessity has helped me develop some good strategies: classrooms that always capture the morning sun as they are a little warmer; heat bags of all types; big coats with warm pockets; and teaching with computers where the warmth generated from top of the processing unit can be very effective.

I have students who readily take my roll, write on the board for me, and turn the heating on in a classroom even before turning on a light. Most importantly, I have had the chance to educate students not only about Raynaud's phenomenon and scleroderma, but also about being different, and accepting it.

Catherine Griffin
Quebec, Canada

It really started to go bad for me in November of 1999. I work on rural mail delivery in Quebec, Canada, and our winters can be quite cold. I had always had cold feet and hands, but this particular winter seemed to have been a lot harder. My hands were swollen all the time and very painful when cold.

By February of 2000, I had to stop working and my family doctor sent me to a rheumatologist in March. By then my right hand was hard as rock. When he told me I had scleroderma, I had no idea what it was. Through family, friends, and the Internet, I came to learn all about it.

Not knowing which type of scleroderma I had was a little scary. From my symptoms, I figured out that it was either CREST or diffuse scleroderma. Because of our hospital's pressure tactics, the test I needed to confirm what type of scleroderma I had could not be done. In September, my test was finally done and came out negative.

In the meantime, I have been going to a skin specialist for treatments with natural products, and it has been working great. In the past two months, I have gone from not being able to hold a knife to peeling potatoes. I have been back at work since April, but I am not sure for how long since winter is just around the corner.

Update – January 2001

Compared to last year, my life has made a complete turnaround because of the fine treatments I have been getting.

I am doing extremely well even though it is the coldest time of the year. I even stopped some of my medication and have cut down on the number of treatments I receive. For those of you who see no hope ahead, this is good news! Chin up!

◆ ❖ ◆

Debbie Dover
Georgia, USA

Here is a copy of the letter I sent to my rheumatologist seeking answers. I have seen this doctor three times since my diagnosis. So far, I have heard nothing back from him.

Dear Doctor,

Thank you for taking the time to call me back last week. Unfortunately, we were not able to connect. I wanted to talk with you about some of the symptoms I have been experiencing. I decided that it may be prudent to write you a short letter outlining these symptoms and to tell you a little about my medical background, because you really do not have that much information. I know your time is valuable and I thank you in advance for taking the time to review this letter. I chose to write this with the hope of improving my current situation and possibly getting answers to some of my questions.

I have had the symptoms of Raynaud's phenomenon for nine years. It started after I was hospitalized for nonspecific uterine bleeding. Up to that point, I had never been sick. Even as a child I was pretty healthy. After the bleeding, which they say may have been caused by a ruptured cyst, things have not been quite the same with my body. I have had a dull pressure and, at times, pain under my left rib ever since. I do not know why, and one of the many physicians I went to said it may be irritable bowel syndrome (IBS). Sometimes the pressure moves to my back and it feels hot. This past week, it was like that and accompanied by headache and vomiting. It might have been caused by a bug, but everything was happening at one time.

During the past six months, I have had at least four very intense headaches accompanied by vomiting. They feel like very bad hangovers. (I remember one from college.) When I get like this, I usually have to stay in bed all day. I was like this for two days this past week, on Tuesday and Saturday. I wondered if it was the medications or a bug.

This past week, I noticed some pain in my jaw (ear area on the right side). It is rather dull, but there is also some discomfort on the left side under my chin and it goes down almost to my collarbone on the left side of my neck. There is a swollen lymph node on the left side of my neck. Sometimes it is bothersome.

The other most notable change is in my thinking. It seems that I have become so much slower in my thinking. I do not know if it is depression and I need something for it or if this disease is affecting my brain. I have told you about the pressure and dizziness. It comes and goes. The best way I can describe it is the way one gets when they cannot sleep and the mind is going one hundred miles an hour. I get like that and I cannot think straight. It is really maddening. I have always been very sharp and on top of things. I would like to know if something is wrong with me medically.

Right before I came to see you in November, I visited a therapist as a last resort. I had been feeling so badly for nine years and thought maybe it was mental since the doctors had treated me that way and could not come up with a diagnosis or reason for my pain. I had never been to a therapist in my life, but I thought, "I have got to change my life." After seeing me twice, he suggested I get a referral to a neurologist to be tested for Multiple Sclerosis (MS). I told him about various symptoms: double vision; dizziness; mental confusion; inability to think straight; numbness in hands, feet, and legs; tingling; Raynaud's phenomenon; fingers locking up on me on the left hand; and pain on left side. To date, no testing for MS has been done, but when my general practitioner heard this he decided to do the antinuclear antibodies (ANA) panel. Then I was told I had CREST. At first I was relieved and felt, at last, my symptoms have been validated. But now I find myself wondering what is happening to me. It is frightening.

Over the past couple of years, I have noticed diminished mental ability. I do not remember things as easily. I can read something and not remember any of it. There are times when I do not recognize things for a couple of seconds. It is really weird. To a degree, it has affected the way I interact with others. I am afraid I am going to have one of these episodes when I am doing something really important. I just need to know what I can do about this and whether or not scleroderma is affecting my mental abilities. Can it?

Do you happen to know what is causing the itching? I am taking the medication, and it has helped me a great deal, but why is it happening in the first place? Should I see an allergist?

I have mentioned the tightness in my chest and the feeling of restricted airflow. I have also noticed discomfort on the left side above my heart. Could this be the esophageal dysfunction?

As for other symptoms, the headaches are the worst aside from the confusion. The tingling and numbness comes and goes in my hands, feet, and legs. Note that it is not accompanied by color changes. I feel some discomfort where a lymphoma was removed from my left arm in 1995.

That just about covers it. I am greatly concerned about some of these things and would like to know if it is just part of the disease. If it is, then I will learn to deal with it. My concern, though, is that I do not want something to go undetected that could be corrected. If it cannot be corrected, I just want to know what I am up against.

Thanks again for your time and I hope to hear from you.

Symptoms: Dizziness; light-headedness; confusion; pressure in head; pressure and pain under the left rib (sometimes more intense, it burns and gets very hot); headaches and nausea; lymph node in neck swollen and slightly tender; tired all the time. Lately, my sleep has been affected somewhat. I wake up very hot and almost sweaty, but then I am okay within a couple of minutes. I wake up at least four to five times a night; I have chest discomfort on the left side above my heart. Sometimes I feel my pulse beating heavily in my temple and neck (left side), tingling in fingers, feet, and legs, and some cramping in calf muscles and fingers.

Six months ago while paddling my kayak, the fingers on my left hand locked up, and I had to pry them open (maybe my fingers were tired, but I had been kayaking regularly for two years without this ever happening). I have not been in a boat but one time since then. I have blurred vision. Nail beds still show broken blood vessels, and the skin on my fingers feels a little tighter.

After summing up my story, I am still angry, still sick, and still confused. I'd like to thank everyone who has answered my questions and shared their stories. It has truly been a big help.

Update – March 2002

Since I posted my story, several people have contacted me to learn more about my condition, while others simply emailed to wish me well. I want to let everyone know that I am much better than I was when I originally posted my story.

I have good days and bad days like anyone, but I am functioning quite well. In 1999, I was scared about my future and this disease called scleroderma. Now I understand it much better, and I know that, to a degree, I can change the way I feel.

It was quite difficult to get to where I am because emotionally, I was a wreck. However, when I learned to accept and understand my condition, I was able to develop a more positive and healthy attitude.

In the beginning, part of my problem was adjusting to the side effects of prescription medications and accepting the fact that I have a degenerative condition. It is not easy to accept at first, but it gets better if you have supportive family, friends, and coworkers. I am blessed in this area.

I have joint and nerve pain, chest pains, irritable bowels, headaches, and Raynaud's phenomenon attacks. Some days my entire hand turns blue! I get through it though. Now these symptoms are part of my daily routine.

If you have been recently diagnosed and you are going through the frightening adjustment phase, perhaps reading how my situation turned around might give you hope.

Debra Hancock
England

One day in 1986, I noticed the index finger on my right hand was continuously cold, as if I had an elastic band around it. This carried on for the next two weeks, until I went to my doctor about something else and just happened to mention this. He was not interested in the illness I had gone to see him about, but he looked very concerned about my finger. He arranged for me to see a consultant that same day.

The consultant examined my finger thoroughly and said there was no pulse in the end of my finger. He presumed I had a blood clot in the finger. For the next twelve months or so, I underwent every test imaginable; I even had an endoscopy. They thought I may have had a blood clot elsewhere and a bit had broken off and traveled to my finger.

Eventually they said they did not think it was anything important, that I should stop smoking and everything would be fine. When I saw my consultant again, my finger had started ulcerating, and a couple of other fingers started doing the same. They ran more tests and eventually, I had a diagnosis of CREST.

The consultant explained it to me briefly, but implied it was not too much to worry about. However, four years before this, I had been referred to the same hospital for an ulcer on my toe, and pain and swelling in my wrists. The consultant at that time also said there was nothing wrong with me. He put it all down to stress, and I left the hospital in tears. I have since been told these were symptoms of CREST.

For many years I have suffered with stomach problems and migraines, and I have only recently found out they are all connected. I have acid reflux. I had Helicobacter pylori, a stomach ulcer, and a hiatal hernia. Although I have been under the same hospital's care for all these problems, nobody linked it to the CREST.

I stopped seeing my consultant three years ago because I was not getting any treatment except aspirin, and I was not made aware of the seriousness of my complaint. Recently, I started suffering with severe stomach pain, and I went to see my local general practitioner (GP). I also told him I had what I call 'blood spots' on my lips and hands, and a large lump in my thumb that kept coming and going. He referred me for yet another endoscopy. He also startled me by saying, "What do you expect? You have CREST, which is a progressively worsening condition."

It was then that everything added up, that I did not have several different conditions; rather, they were all part of CREST. The lump in my thumb is Calcinosis, the 'C' in CREST. I already knew I had Raynaud's phenomenon, which is the 'R' in CREST. All my stomach complaints are esophagealrelated, the 'E' in CREST., and the blood spots are telangiectasia, the "T" in CREST.

I also have many other complaints, which after reading information on the Internet, I believe may be related. I keep getting boils everywhere, and I seem to have at least two at any one time. My GP has referred me back to my consultant, at my request, and I will not leave the hospital until I am fully aware of what to expect in the future.

What surprises me was that four years ago, I had a cold finger and was told it probably would not get any worse. Now I have nearly all the symptoms of CREST, and I worry what the future holds. I am only thirty-four years old and have two sons, ages fourteen and sixteen, and a daughter age three. Will the CREST stop me from being the kind of mum I want to be?

I have so many questions. I have read on the Internet that people die from this condition. Will that happen to me? Each day I hope my symptoms will not get worse, but when so much has happened in four years, I do not feel very positive.

I recently went to the dentist with a severe toothache. The dentist refused to treat me for a root filling because he did not understand CREST. I had to wait another three weeks to be treated and even then, a different dentist had to do it because the original one was still unsure.

Nobody understands when you explain the condition. If you have asthma, multiple sclerosis (MS), or any other well-known condition, if you tell people about it, they understand. They will help carry your bags or will not allow you to do things that are detrimental to your health. However, try explaining to someone that you have CREST and would they mind doing this for you, and they think you are a hypochondriac (which I have been called many times, even by my own family).

People just see the outside. I look like a reasonably fit young woman, so why should anyone help me? Even my own partner does not understand. Just last week, he asked me to hold our daughter's ice-lolly because she did not want it and he was driving. I tried to explain it could damage my fingers and he looked at me as if I was stupid. I just hope the consultant I see will give me the answers I am looking for and give me a little hope.

◆ ❖ ◆

Denise Such
England

It all started when I was sixteen years old. I was having awful pains in my hands and feet. The doctor said it was rheumatism. This went on for years. It got worse and I had other symptoms like white, then purple, then red hands; it was the same with my feet. My legs hurt, and I was having trouble with my thyroid.

I was sent to a specialist who ran some tests that came back negative. I was told to take painkillers when needed and maybe come back when I was fifty and something might show up then. I was really upset and could not believe the attitude of this so-called doctor. I went home in tears.

I was twenty-eight by then, and I really could not take anymore. I was tired all the time, I hurt all over, my hands and feet were going a bit out of shape, and the pain was unbearable. I went to see another doctor who told me I was just depressed and gave me antidepressants. Although the pills made me relax a little, it still did not explain my symptoms.

At last I saw a new general practitioner (GP) who actually listened to me, did every test possible, and then sent me to see Professor Cooper. What a relief! Dr. Cooper took great interest and, as a result, diagnosed me with Raynaud's phenomenon and CREST. As it is a hard disease to understand, I felt that at least someone was listening to the pain I had suffered for years. I felt no one believed me, as if I was making it all up.

Five years ago, I became really sick, lost weight, and could not eat. After being admitted to the hospital, it showed my liver had been affected. This showed I had systemic sclerosis. I spent seven weeks in the hospital.

Three months later, swallowing became difficult, and my large bowel became affected. I spent another five weeks in the hospital, but at least I was being looked after.

I am now on fifteen different medications. I do not really know what or how I would do without the medication or without my GP, Dr. Cooper, and his associate, Karen.

I am forty-five now, and although I suffered for years, I have come to terms with the disease and accepted it, which is hard to do. Unfortunately, I must have an ileostomy as my large bowel refuses to work, but I am positive I will cope.

I have a supportive husband and siblings, and my elderly parents are very caring. I have two boys, ages thirty and twenty-five, who unfortunately will not accept what I have, but we are working on it. I have three lovely granddaughters, and they help me along and give me a reason to get up in the morning.

I have good days and bad days. I have not worked in four years and I do miss this. I was an auxiliary nurse for sixteen years. I used to look after others, and now they have to look after me. I found the isolation very hard to cope with, but our true friends will always be there. I now have an email friend, who I contacted through this web site, and that is great. Keep warm, everyone, and take care.

Donald A. Alfera
With Service Dog Brandy
Washington, USA

I entitle this *My Time So Far with Scleroderma* because this has been a journey unlike any I could ever imagine in my life. I would like to share some of my personal experiences over the past six years.

I have been married for twenty-six years to a very loving lady named Karolynne. We have two children who are both married, and two grandchildren of our eldest child and his wife. As for my service dog, Brandy, I will introduce her in good time.

I enlisted in the United States Navy in 1972, went into submarine duty, and spent my first hitch serving on what is called a Fast Attack submarine, which is a submarine without a missile platform. During that time I traveled over much of the Atlantic Ocean and even under the ice up north. I left the service when my father died and stayed in the reserves for the next few years.

During this time, I lived in my hometown of Mechanicsburg, Pennsylvania. Most people who are old enough might remember this famous town where the Three Mile Island Nuclear Power Plant incident occurred. I met Karolynne there and she was part of most of my teen years. She and I shared the same friends and most of the same activities. We married and started our family. I bring all this up as some people look for relationships between scleroderma and life experiences. I do not feel the exposure to the air or any potential steam leaks from the nuclear plant were contributing factors to my later diagnosed illness.

We decided, as a family, to re-enlist in the active Navy to finish my career. My career was filled with duty stations around the world on each kind of submarine, except the deep submergence project boats. Shore duty took me to the Indian Ocean, all over the United States, and to the outer reaches of the Alaskan Islands. My career was ended before I was ready, because my illness began to develop in mid-1990.

I was serving onboard a submarine in the Pacific Northwest, and the first symptoms were severe reflux and early temperature sensitivities. Naturally, being a healthy person, the doctors prescribed an antacid and told me to let go of some of the stress. I took antacid to the point where I had a bottle everywhere I went and just drank it as I needed, which was quite often. Finally, the doctor decided they needed to have a closer look at what was going on. The internist, who saw me at the time, stated that I had Barrett's esophagus with a hernia. I also had gallstones.

During 1994 and 1995, I had one surgery after another: polyps removed from my vocal chords; gallbladder removed; and a procedure called Nissen fundoplication, where the stomach is moved around the esophagus to form an additional flap to keep the acid down. The doctors were amazed all this was going on simultaneously. They also discovered pleural thickening, restrictive in nature, in my lungs, and thickening of my bladder.

These two years were difficult. In the military, you were not supposed to be sick and if you were, you were considered broken. Many times, superior officers wanted me to leave the service because anything more than a broken bone or something they could not see made no sense to them, so they thought I must have been exaggerating the situation or dragging it out.

The military leaders who praised my work for twenty years were turning against my career status. Karolynne and I were just holding on, trying to get through one new diagnosis at a time. Our children were simply lost wondering what was happening to their father. I decided to take as many medications as I needed and say I was feeling fine.

At this point, I took a position at a small Navy facility on the Indian Ocean called Diego Garcia. The job was demanding, but I was away from family, all home-life stress, and the time off work was always filled with warm weather, a warm-water lagoon on the island in which to swim, and Tosca, a new partner, became my best friend. By this time, my joints and hands were becoming more sensitive to the cold, the gastrointestinal problems were getting worse, and to top it all off, I was experiencing my first real bouts with fatigue.

Tosca was a Royal Air Force drug detection dog. He and I had spent many hours checking all food and shipping containers, as well as flights that contained food for drugs or other contraband. Then Tosca developed a seizure condition that resulted in mandatory retirement.

Tosca and I were in the same boat. I could not let the medical people know what was going on because it would land me back in the States and by this time, Tosca and I were quite close. He now lived in the barracks with me. I learned to chart his seizures, administer his medications, and properly exercise and care for him. The American Military chain of command wanted him destroyed, as he could no longer work. Even though Tosca had been given his rabies shots on the island, he could not return home to the UK, which is a rabies-free country.

Somehow I knew this was the real attitude: If you no longer fit the needs of those who pull the strings, you were useless. As my condition worsened, the pressure to have Tosca put down increased. To my advantage, this was a U.S. Navy facility, but this was a British-owned island and they had the upper hand. The British would not allow him to be destroyed. This fact is important because it was my first fight—and Alamo!

In fighting for what I believed, scleroderma cost me my career. An illness does not make me useless. I could see myself in what this wonderful four-year-old Labrador was going through.

When my tour of duty on the island was over, and under the shelter of his status as a British working dog, I brought Tosca home with me halfway around the world. Once home, I could hide things no longer. I was tripping over my feet on tile floors, needed naps throughout the day, and I had my first main outward sign—a skin plaque I could not hide from Karolynne. I had a biopsy and then my world started to change. I now had a doctor say the word scleroderma. Wow, so much to learn, so much to do. Of course, I read all I could. I hit the libraries and the Internet, and that's why 1995 was a year I will never forget.

I learned that doctors did not know much and that they did not agree much on what they did know. Researchers were not in agreement, so, of course, regular doctors did not know what to think. I was fortunate enough to find a family doctor who asked me what I wanted to do. I was confused and, to paraphrase, he said, "We can fight the symptoms or we can study you for development like a lab rat."

He had treated several people during his tour in Japan and was familiar with treatment, testing procedures, and protocols. He was wonderful at helping me find information and learn to make decisions about my own care and treatment plan. Other doctors were fighting and changing the diagnosis, but they never left the word scleroderma out of the conversation. I had a doctor who was willing to be proactive.

This doctor put a stop to my military chain of command's attempt to put me out. He helped me start my treatment and plan for a retirement with which I could feel comfortable. After serving twenty-three years, I did not deserve to be tossed aside like an old newspaper. I had earned the right to maintain my dignity and respect for a proper retirement. Thanks to this doctor, I was able to gain just that.

In October of 1996, I retired from the military. Then I learned the nightmare of dealing with the Veterans Administration and with Social Security Disability. I also learned this illness was not going to get better or just go away. With the help of some wonderful people, other patients, and my loving wife, we found a way to take one step at a time to work through this new system.

I have since developed hypertension, pulmonary fibrosis, Sjögren's Syndrome, and an assortment of other natural progressions. I cannot stand the heat for it makes it harder to breathe and my skin itches like crazy. I cannot stand the cold, as my hands and feet will take on a new color scheme.

I have learned that having esophageal dilation every now and then is not so bad; it actually keeps me swallowing with a fairly normal feeling. The twenty to thirty pills I take each day, everything from blood thinners to antidepressants, diuretics to blood pressure medications, are just part of my day. Pain seems to be a part of my day, but I am getting better at dealing with it and decreasing the pain medications, except on the worst of days.

Karolynne and I have learned that today is the most important day of our lives, and we have the future planned as best we can. Now we think of things like travel, friends, and spending time with each other, our kids, grandchildren, and, of course, our dogs.

I did lose my friend Tosca, but only in the physical sense. The lessons he helped me learn about life, such as finding the inner strength to stand up for what I believe and not compromising at the expense of my value system—lessons like that are priceless. Many mornings after I wake from a short nap, all four of my dogs are on the bed all around me with my Brandy resting her head on my chest just looking up at me. They keep me safe and continue to show me the value of giving to others, understanding how important it is to never lose myself in the heat of the moment or in the middle of the battle.

I have trained three dogs that are now fully qualified for service work. Karol and I are currently training two more wonder black Labradors.

Karol has retired from working for many years and raising our sons while I was gone to sea or other places around the world. Now we have time to share all the wonderful things this life has to offer.

I am not sad or resentful of this illness or of the physical things I have experienced. Those are not important to me; they are but a small part of what this life has to offer. I am very thankful for the opportunity to learn who I really am. I know what my value system truly is; I believe in what I stand for. I'm thankful for the forty-seven years I have lived. I have lived them to the maximum. After all, many years ago, I never thought I would live past thirty, so now I am in bonus rounds.

I close with a favorite quote from a movie that has impacted my life for many years: "Live, live, live! Life is a banquet and most poor suckers are starving to death!" I will never say, "If only."

Jenny C. Besaw
Florida, USA

I was just diagnosed with severe CREST syndrome one week ago. Since the diagnosis, I have started to educate myself about scleroderma in order to understand what I need to do to help control and manage my condition. The first few days I projected a lot of different outcomes, including my death (I hope this is normal.). The words the doctor spoke that day kept ringing in my head, "Some people have died from this disease." The ringing did not last very long once I started thinking about my twelve-year-old son, who I have raised on my own for the past eight years.

This disease has taken part of my right index finger and nearly the right middle finger. The ulcerations are bad and very painful. The first episode, eight years ago, was never linked to scleroderma. My symptoms started to appear over ten years ago, but I was only recently diagnosed. I was referred to many different doctors for complaints over the years. None of them ever put it all together.

I have all five CREST symptoms. The good news is that the battery of tests and X rays show no internal organ involvement at this time. As a runner who completed one full marathon and recently the Disney half, it is so hard for me to believe I have this chronic lifelong disease.

Update – March 2002

It has been one year since my diagnosis of severe CREST syndrome with limited scleroderma. I have skin thickening on the hands, facial area, and feet. I would like to share my successes and my setbacks. I have learned so much and become more educated about this disease. This statement sounds funny because I consider myself a very educated woman. I hold both a B.S. and an M.S. in Management Information Systems, but that is not the kind of education that helped me through the past year.

This disease is so individualized and can rear its head when you least expect it. The best education to help me has come from all of you and from my doctors, who have strived to find the best ways possible to manage my symptoms.

Now I am learning how to prevent Raynaud's phenomenon attacks, not attacks from computer viruses. I am fighting fatigue when I just want to sleep all day, not a slow and poor-performing network. I am adjusting my diet to prevent painful and erosive acid reflux, not fixing the abnormal termination of a computer program.

I am still a runner. It is a personal hobby that brings me great joy, but this disease has taken some of that away. I completed my last marathon in January. On the advice of my doctors, I will not continue to run such long distances.

I will, however, continue moderate exercise and a positive attitude. I pray every day that a cure is found and the suffering ends. I read your stories and hear your voices and this, in itself, provides strength.

Juanita "Jackie" Vasselin
Georgia, USA

I was diagnosed over twenty years ago, and if my sister did not have the same symptoms as me, I never would have known about scleroderma. We were identical twins, and she died in 1988 from kidney failure. We had the same genes; we both started with Raynaud's phenomenon.

By the time my sister was diagnosed, she was pretty involved with it. Her organs failed fast. As for me, at first my hands got worse, although I am lucky that I have not had ulcers. I had dry skin, swallowing was difficult, and I was short of breath at the time.

It was not until 1997 that I was diagnosed with pulmonary hypertension (PH). I had an episode in the hospital yard, and they rushed me right into the emergency room. The next day, they transported me to a hospital in Atlanta, Georgia, for a heart catheter. They discovered the PH at that time. I am on oxygen twenty-four/seven. I have no energy, and my breathing has gotten worse. I live one day at a time because I never know how I will feel when I get up.

I have a very good friend who helps me a lot. My family tells me not to overdo—or do, period. I cook, and go to the store and to church. Things are not always easy, but at least I am here to write to all of you. I enjoy my computer as you are my entire world.

Judy Rose Thompson
New Hampshire, USA

I was originally diagnosed with CREST in 1991. It has since been upgraded to systemic sclerosis. Looking back, my first symptoms occurred in 1974, two years after giving birth to my daughter. I had gangrene in two fingers, pneumonia, and all kinds of weird infections. Prior to that, I had always had irritable bowels; I have never been regular. Raynaud's phenomenon was also present.

Four years later, I had a hysterectomy due to endometriosis and have never felt right since then. Most doctors told me it was stress or all in my head, so the frustration turned inward. I was severely depressed for years, mostly because I was always tired and physically miserable, but since the doctors had found nothing specific, I also blamed myself and even had one suicide attempt.

Finally, due to a severe esophageal stricture (I was down to one hundred pounds because it hurt to eat and swallow) and severe chest pain, my daughter rushed me to the emergency room thinking I was having a heart attack. There I met the doctor who saved my life. After undergoing testing for AIDS, leukemia, multiple sclerosis (MS), and a list of other possibilities, he told me I have CREST/scleroderma—which I had never heard of, nor had anyone else I knew. He also said, "One in two hundred people gets a disease in their lifetime, and scleroderma is like having twenty to thirty diseases at once." That made my day.

After that, I went through the disability process and moved back home with my parents. The loss of my independence has been the hardest thing, but after a few years of heavy-duty soul searching and major adjustments, I am happy and look at my disease as a blessing in disguise.

I have since written three novels. *The Kiss of Judas* was published in 1996. Publishers are considering the other two. I have made good use of all this free time, and I think that is the secret. Keep busy, even if it is just reading or surfing the Internet.

Update – February 2002

Since I published my story on the website over a year ago, I have received several uplifting and supportive emails, which I have surely appreciated. I also lost a dear friend, Julie, to scleroderma. She was the first other scleroderma person I ever met in person!

My daughter is showing early signs (Raynaud's phenomenon) of this disease.

I write now with encouragement that life indeed does go on! I recently published my second novel, *A Switch in Time*. It is a historical, spiritual, and futuristic adventure story where one of my main characters gets scleroderma. I thought that it would be a good way to give this disease some much-needed exposure as it still astounds me how many medical and regular people have never heard of scleroderma.

My message today is that anything is possible, sick or not sick. We are not our bodies. Keep the faith everyone! Please look at this disease—or any disease—as a gift, a blessing in disguise. Our downtime can be just what we have been praying for to tackle some of our dreams!

Laurie Schonert
California, USA

I am forty-nine years old. I have been happily married to my high school sweetheart for almost thirty-one years. We have two grown, beautiful and successful daughters and the greatest gift of a granddaughter.

My first symptoms of this disorder began with Raynaud's phenomenon when I was in my mid twenties. We used to think it was funny how my fingers would turn purple in the shower, then red and white in the most amazing, colorful display. At that time, I saw a physician who said I might have lupus or scleroderma. My mom was constantly being tested for lupus at that same time.

One doctor to the next could not seem to agree, but I knew about lupus. What I read about scleroderma did not seem to apply to me. The doctor said there was really no treatment available. As I had no medical insurance, I opted not to pay for the tests. The advice from reading about this disease was to quit smoking and move to a warmer climate. Because I have never had a cigarette in my life and lived in the desert, I figured that was all I could do for myself.

Once I understood what arterial spasms were, I decided they were not good for me and kept myself reasonably warmer in an effort to prevent them. Typical arthritis-like complaints accompanied my Raynaud's phenomenon, but otherwise, I was doing okay.

I continued my life as a Jazzercise instructor. My daughters got involved in figure skating, and then keeping myself warm became more difficult. I had one bad season with fingertip ulcers, and another physician said I probably had scleroderma. That is as far as the discussions went.

I later became a teacher and between ice skating and teaching, our family life was busy. I had some sort of nuisance disease that, just barely, slowed me down.

About eight years ago, our life was complicated with a move to a new mountain community to assist in advancing my skaters. We lived and trained ice-skating in Lake Arrowhead, California.

Eventually, the stress of the competitive ice-skating as well as the residence and job change really took its toll on me. The Raynaud's phenomenon was really bad by then. I had good medical insurance, so my new doctor pushed forward to identify and treat my condition.

I was definitively diagnosed with CREST, with the C, R, E, and T all clearly present. The antinuclear antibodies (ANA) tests, clearly and repeatedly, suggested CREST.

The aching joints and muscle fatigue were my next symptoms, followed by degenerative spine disorder, a herniated disc, difficulty breathing, and chest pains. My doctor tried to treat everything at once and was actually quite successful at it. Although my blood pressure is low, high blood pressure medicine helped with the Raynaud's phenomenon. Physical therapy and anti-inflammatories helped with the pain. Lung function tests came out okay. My cardiac tests showed good arterial flow, but they also revealed damaged sections of my heart, specifically, the damaged anterior left ventricle and non-reactive septum.

The cardiologist casually said it must have been from my heart attack to which I vehemently replied that I had never had any heart attacks. He thought I was just a silly girl, who did not know her own body, but fortunately, my general practitioner (GP) was a listener, a thinker, and a problem-solver.

Three years ago, some superficial blood clots lead to two pulmonary embolisms and my doctor had a hard time convincing the specialists they had actually occurred. Surgery on my leg to clean out the clots seemed to go well. About two weeks later, I was rushed to the emergency room. A series of weeks in various hospitals got me out of danger and on blood thinners, which I still take to this day.

Trips to have my esophagus dilated have become routine, and I take all the GERD medicines to try to prevent further damage.

I suffered a debilitating depression that knocked me out of reality for a while following my hospital stays, but medication and an uncommonly supportive family and friends got me through. I do not know how my husband and daughters have held up so well. This condition of mine has put us all through some hard times. God bless Taylor, my little red-haired angel, as she can always make me smile.

I have had help from too many people to mention, but they are all part of where I am today. I can still work, and I love teaching high school biology. Sometimes I get way too tired to function, but everyone involved with me seems to understand.

Currently, I take many medications, as appropriate. Being a well-informed patient and keeping track of all my own conditions, treatments, and current complaints, helps my doctors.

I am tired a lot lately and am experiencing serious problems with intestinal motility, which a specialist is investigating.

My biggest concerns are for my loved ones and their health. My sister has fibromyalgia and lymphoma. My mother has battled the typical autoimmune nightmare of not having a clear diagnosis of anything but arthritis and a lot of questions. My oldest daughter has unexplained rashes and joint pain, while my youngest has psoriatic rheumatoid arthritis and is currently being tested for ankylosing spondylitis. She had to quit ice-skating due to the pain. Although our diagnoses are all different, they all seem to be autoimmune related.

I enjoy every day that I'm gifted, and I am eternally grateful for the love shared with me by so many. It sounds crazy, but in many ways this horrible disease has been one of my life's greatest blessings.

Thanks for reading my story. Maybe it will help someone else.

Lorrie Ann Moses
Louisiana, USA

Hi, my name is Lorrie. I am twenty-six years old and was diagnosed with limited scleroderma/CREST in February 2002. My symptoms started around November of 1996. There were ulcerations on my fingertips, and I had severe heartburn.

By the latter part of 1998, I had begun having severe stomach problems. I was always vomiting, and the heartburn was so bad that I could not sleep lying down.

In June 1999, when I began having problems swallowing, I decided it was time to see a doctor. But before I did, I found out I was pregnant. I had a normal pregnancy with no problems at all.

My daughter was born in June 2000. After her birth, I went to the doctor about my swallowing problem. I was told I had a stricture caused from acid reflux.

In January of 2001, the stricture was dilated. In February, I began having the problem again. The doctors said it was normal and dilated the stricture a second time in July. I was put on medication for it, and I have had no problems since.

In August, I noticed red spots on my lips and hard spots on my elbows. In October, I went to a dermatologist about the hard spots on my elbow. He removed them and two weeks later, he told me it was calcinosis and that it was rare, but nothing serious. Before the end of my appointment, I asked him to take a look at my fingers, which I was having problems with, again. He asked me a few questions and referred me to a rheumatologist. After all kinds of tests, I was diagnosed and started on medications.

I am twenty-six years old and feel like a pillhead. I am not sure what to think about all this. At first I thought, "Oh my goodness! I am going to die." But my doctor assured me that I could very likely live to be an old woman.

I am worried about my skin because I do not know what will happen. My fingers really hurt. My elbow still has not healed. I don't feel well at all.

On a good note, summer is almost here! Maybe with the sunlight my fingers will heal along with my elbow. I am hoping and praying for a cure. Thanks for reading my story.

◆ ❖ ◆

Melissa Schonasky
Wisconsin, USA

I am a twenty-eight-year-old single mother of two small children. When I was about fourteen years old, I started having problems with my joints. My parents took me from doctor to doctor. They all agreed I had some sort of arthritic problem, but they did not know what it was.

As I got older, I started to experience pain and sensitivity to cold in my fingers and toes. My doctor said it must be poor circulation due to my smoking habit and told me to quit. Of course, as a rebellious teen, I was having none of that.

I just kept visiting different doctors and doing most of what they told me to do. My mother kept asking for answers. Some doctors told her it was probably all in my head. After all, each appointment got me out of school for a while. I swear there is nothing like knowing something is wrong with you only to be told you are being overly dramatic.

After the birth of my second child at age twenty-four, I really started to have problems. I had trouble walking at times, I was cold, and I had constant heartburn. I was also afraid I would drop my beautiful new baby because I just did not seem to have any strength.

Once again, I headed to the family doctor's office thinking I would be told to rest, take vitamins, quit smoking—in short, get a life and stop bothering them about this.

This time was different. Recently, I had started seeing a new, younger doctor who seemed to be pretty open-minded. He took a look at me and asked me in-depth questions, some of which seemed silly to me: "Do you take water to bed with you at night?" Well, of course, doesn't everyone? I thought it was normal. The answer is no, not everyone takes water to bed with them.

After asking me about fifty questions, I still thought some of them were silly. He asked me to wash off my makeup. At this point, I was thinking this man has to be off his rocker. I knew he was off his rocker when he commented on the red veins and blotches on my face. Didn't everyone have them? I always thought that was why women plastered their faces. Hmmm, guess not!

He drew blood, and the results were possible CREST syndrome. Researcher that I am, I decided to look into this before my appointment with a rheumatologist. At that time, the only information I could find was extremely depressing and scary.

The first rheumatologist I saw did not believe there was a problem and insisted on drawing blood. After all, I was so young at the initial onset of my symptoms. The results came back the same. I refused to have anything more to do with the subject and doctors, because I was tired of being told there was nothing wrong with me. I was tired of being a member of the diagnosis-of-the-month club.

About eighteen months ago, things became unbearable again. I went back to the family doctor. He was upset to hear about what happened at my appointment with the rheumatologist and that I was too upset and scared to go back again. He made another appointment for me with a different rheumatologist and insisted I keep it.

Well, I kept the appointment and am happy to say I finally started to get some answers. The answers are not always what I want to hear, but they are answers just the same.

I am sorry to see there are so many other people suffering from this, but I am glad to see that I can now find more than just the scary and depressing information.

Update – September 1999

I want to let you know that since I posted my story, I have gotten responses from many people. I feel better knowing I am not alone, and that I now have other people with whom to communicate. Thank you!

◆❖◆

Pamela Anne Harris
Victoria, Australia

I have big hugs for Pat, my twin sister. She is my medicine without drugs, my laughter, my hands, and my helper. When she feels my pain, she will take a four-hour trip with no complaints.

My story began in 1972. This part is relevant to my diagnosis. Five months after my marriage broke down, my ex-husband took my seven-year-old son from the babysitter while I was at work. Within days he allowed him to cross a busy highway. My son was struck and killed instantly.

I was completely shattered and unable to attend his burial. Pat laid six long-stemmed red roses on his little white coffin.

I began a daily routine of injections and medication. Life was a complete blur. A doctor was treating me for arthritis and my whole body ached. I became allergic to many drugs: antibiotics, penicillin, and cortisone.

One year later, I was no better. My skin, as well as being blotchy, became very tight and my fingers had open wounds continuously. I could not raise my arms above my shoulders.

Through friends at my workplace (animal nutritional research), I took the advice of a research scientist and sought a second opinion. The new doctor took a long look at my hands and consulted with his colleague. Then an appointment was made for me to visit a dermatologist.

This became the longest day of my life. My mind went blank when the specialist took only seconds, then asked me to lie down because he had some bad news. A word was mentioned as he began to explain my rare condition that, according to records, I would be about the twelfth case diagnosed in Australia.

All I could say was, "Am I dying?" I vaguely heard: "Two years at the most. Within three months, you will be wheelchair bound. There is no cure." My only thought was, "How can I tell my only son that I was going to die so soon after his brother?"

The doctor rattled on about the reason for my complaints. I still did not know the name of this horrid disease; it had yet to register in my mind. He said he believed it was caused by a severe emotional upset.

I was admitted to the hospital and went through traumatic tests. Several weeks later I was allowed to leave the hospital with a letter and a prescription. I opened the letter. It was from my work. It said that due to my illness, I was unable to return to my duties.

The next day I forced myself to go to my workplace. I had the name of my complaint written down and I gave it to one of the animal research scientists. That is when it all started happening. He immediately did a lot of reading and came to me with a bottle of vitamin E. I took his advice and began taking massive doses.

Within three months I was walking back into the hospital. The doctors were amazed. They patted me on the back. Examinations proved that the disease had arrested at my knees. I thank my office staff for all the time they put into pushing me around on a bike, and also for the Gene Pitney and Village People tapes to which they made me dance every morning, afternoon, and during lunch breaks.

Each weekend, I went dancing. I was so concerned because I did not want to end up in a wheelchair. I then had all my mobility back in my lower legs, although the pain in other parts of my body was very severe.

My son went on through his schooling. He began an apprenticeship as a cabinetmaker. I decided to further my studies with a poultry husbandry course. Studying played a little minor havoc with me. Studying with little rest became stressful, not that I would ever admit it at that stage of my life. I was still not taking any medication for scleroderma, but was carrying on, watching my diet intake of heaps of fruits and vegetables and vitamin E capsules. In 1980-1981, my son was sent away to the country on a job that was quite a distance from me and was unable to come home daily.

Unfortunately, I suffered a muscular breakdown. Unable to move from my bed, I laid for four days without food or water. I was on leave from my work, so no one was aware. Suddenly, my son walked in the door. My prayers had been answered. His place of employment had run out of timber on-site. To this day, I ask myself how they picked him over everyone else to come back with the truck driver. My son quickly called a doctor and I was admitted to the hospital suffering from malnutrition. I was "saved by the bell," so to speak. I sat in the hospital with an IV drip for three weeks.

When I was stronger, I was able to finish my final exam paper in my poultry husbandry class with triple A's! I went on to do a computer business course.

You can never give up, no matter what; this is strictly my opinion. I have been acknowledged in many animal research papers, and I have assisted animal research scientists with experiments that have been published in various journals. I did seventeen years of judging at the Royal Melbourne Show for poultry exhibits.

I also was hired for a higher position with full-time office duties, and during the last six years I was the finance officer for the Department of Agriculture in the animal research unit. After twenty-four years, I retired from this position in June 1992. Prior to this, I had joined the research unit for scleroderma at the Royal Melbourne Hospital.

The little and middle fingers on my left hand had severely deformed. They had curled inward, with the fingernails embedded into my palm. When this occurred, the bone on the little finger protruded through the skin, causing gangrene. I had a prostaglandin infusion and amputation, leaving a small stump on my little finger, and a partial amputation of my middle finger knuckle. That was in August of 1992. The prostaglandin infusion was a great success, and my wounds healed very quickly. Since then, I have had several amputations.

I became bored and took up arts and crafts with the aid of my friend, Sue, and I started going to markets each weekend. But the cold got to me as Raynaud's phenomenon is part of my condition. Because of the cold and poor blood circulation, I feel it caused my other fingers to become infected. In 1995-1996, the tips of my left thumb and ring finger became infected. The soft tissue area was very painful. I withstood the pain as long as I could and then decided to have my second operation. With the doctor's advice, the same procedure took place. This left me with only my index finger. It has now curled under what is left of my middle finger.

I became bored again, so I went into the workforce once more as a cashier for another two years. I finally retired for good in November 1999.

I attended the research unit at Royal Melbourne Hospital until the doctors who attended to me went on to further their careers or changed over to the rheumatology department. The doctor who attends to me is the same one from the research unit. I have great faith in this doctor. I had my usual visit to my local general practitioner (GP) in March 2000 for all the normal blood tests, etc. After all these years, I asked him what type of scleroderma I had. His reply: "The worst, but keep doing what you are doing because you are a battler. It could be work, vitamin E, or your positive outlook that has helped."

Scleroderma was an absolutely dreaded word to me. My life expectancy of two years was now twenty-seven years and counting, and I was able to stay in the work force until 1999. I led a near-normal life, keeping a home and seeing my remaining son, Tom, reach manhood and get married to Gillian. Now I am enjoying my grandchildren, Tim and Emily.

Update – May 2000

You have a rundown on my hands. Prior to my operations, I must go through a prostaglandin infusion for seventy-two hours. I fear drips unless they are attached to a monitor. A tube is inserted in the side of my throat, which is directed through my veins to the heart and lung region. I have bolts on both sides of my neck to restrain me (no joke). I am scared from the time of its insertion until its removal without this! I have no healing process, so the prostaglandin dilates my veins for a good blood flow and healing. I was a first for this, and now others have followed.

I am embarrassed to mention some of my internal problems. But what the heck, I am still here. I have no control over my bowel. Each morning I use a mini-enema to clean the bowel out completely and then use a disposable napkin before I leave the house. I had many tests taken for cancer and they were all negative.

Next on the agenda is my swallowing. I am only on baby food and mashed vegetables. Professor Young informed me seven years ago, after one of my annual endoscopes, that he was only able get a baby tube down my throat. He woke me from the land of nod just to tell me this great news. My reply was, "Well, then I will eat baby food!" I am now used to the fact that I am unable to munch an apple or have a big juicy steak. Meat went out of my diet twenty-five years ago.

I have puffing (shortness of breath) from the lung deterioration. I also have a heart rhythm abnormality, found only three years ago, even though I had been complaining about butterflies in my chest from the onset of my diagnosis. I would say they put me through more echocardiograms than all of the heart patients in Australia.

The heart rhythm abnormality was picked up accidentally. When the cardiologist was called to the phone, he asked the nurse to remove the equipment. She asked what was going on. I shook my head, as always, leaving things as they were. She waited for the doctor (and more doctors by this time). I was shaking in my boots lying down, as I was scared out of my wits. My greatest fear ever is of having a heart problem.

I should not worry. My dad was ninety-two when he passed away, and we were told that his heart would not stop beating even after he suffered a major stroke. It took three weeks before he finally gave in. My sister (one out of eight) told him to hurry up or she would beat him to heaven!

I am taking medication for the heart problems. I also have angina and high cholesterol, which is now under control with medication plus the usual diet of no animal fats. For the hiatal hernia, I take a proton pump inhibitor. I have been on this capsule for many years and cannot start the day without it. I take three goblets of water to bed with me each night (I cannot lift a jug.). As soon as I open my eyes, I reach for this capsule. It takes two full goblets for me to swallow it. Within half an hour, my throat feels open and there is no heartburn.

Then I take another tablet that gets my body and muscles on the move. Now I can manage to rise and get myself a mug of coffee, which I take back to bed. After I stop puffing, I sit back and watch the soapies taped the day before. At breakfast, I have another coffee with my bowl of cereal. I rest until mid-morning, either in bed or at the computer, and then it is coffee time again.

I never use medical terms, because people always say, "What?" So the only reference I make is that I have tight skin. I have intense Raynaud's phenomenon and winter is my enemy along with sudden weather changes, which play havoc in the form of vasospasms. Ugh!

I also have alopecia (hair loss), which was caused by an antibiotic. I have hairpieces from short to long and wear three-deep shoulder pads as my shoulders are as round as a ball.

I have calcinosis, which is a buildup of calcium. My general practitioner (GP) tells me that it is not due to too much calcium in my diet. I have large, hard deposits on my fingers and now one on my ankle. At times it oozes out like zinc cream from a tube, and I cannot resist picking and squeezing it—but that habit stopped when the amputations began. To dress my wounds, I clean them with tea tree oil and then apply Savlon powder and a bandage.

Update – August 2000

Once again, I have had another operation. This time the prostaglandin infusion was the worst I ever experienced. It took several hours to insert the line. They attempted four different places in my chest. Once the line was inserted into my jugular vein, all went smoothly for the seventy-two hour procedure. Instead of having general anesthesia, I had an arm block. I was sleepy, but not quite out, so I could not feel it but, golly gee, I could hear it. It took a lot out of me (age catching up—ha ha!). During my hospital stay, I went on oxygen for several hours at a time along with some asthmatic sprays. I heard this crackling sound and was informed that it was coming from my lungs.

They tried to repair the deformed fingers on my right hand. As it turned out, they amputated my index finger to mid-knuckle. This was the one finger that was okay. It was not turned-in or deformed like my others, but it had an infection. The surgeons found that the bone had completely disintegrated to the knuckle. They then removed the mid-knuckles from the three other fingers, leaving me with my thumb as the only finger without surgery. I spent a year dealing with this. I now carry a letter with my identification from my local GP, in case I am ever asked to sign any documents.

Update – September 2001

I developed another muscular breakdown; my fourth. Two of these required hospitalization and IV treatments, unlike the others, which I was able to stay home with oral antibiotics.

Yippee, I can walk again without that darned walker and I am out of bed four to five hours a day again! Stress will never rear its nasty head with me again. I know you all are having problems. Chin up!

Update – January 2002

On January 21, I returned to the hospital to have all my pre-operation tests for further amputations. I also had a urinary tract infection. Could anything else go wrong? Further testing is necessary for treating my bowel, which is rather severe now. In Australia, when you have a disability, you are put on a list for permanent pickups to the hospital by an ambulance.

Seven days later, I was back at the hospital for the results and discussion of the colonoscopy with the specialists. I would need an operation to perform the insertion of a colon bag. After much ado with other specialists, it was decided that due to my amputations, I would be unable to manage the bag. When my caregivers are not on duty, it would be too difficult for me.

Update – February 2002

On February 2, the local GP took a further urine test, which came up negative. Wow! Another plus! These are few and far between.

My rheumatologist assured me a few days later that the colon bag would be of no use. They discussed the possibility that the vein in my left arm looked okay for another prostaglandin infusion. Let us hope so anyway.

On the morning of February 18, I woke up with severe pain in my right elbow. I waited for my caregiver as I was unable to get up from bed. She looked me over and found that my elbow had a huge, red lump the size of a tomato. She found another forming on my backbone to the right of my backside, so she called my local GP. I was prescribed an antibiotic and painkiller. The diagnosis was a bone infection. The pain medicine was only a partial relief, and the antibiotic is slowly working. I have two more days of treatment. I can now move my arm, but am still finding it hard to get out of bed.

I received a letter on February 22 regarding further amputations, which will not take place until I am completely well again. Ha ha! The next prostaglandin infusion is set for April 15, with amputations on April 18, if my infection is all clear. By then, who knows, "I may have more," I say laughing. That is what my life is about. Laughter is medicine.

Please, always think positive, keep your chin up, and smile through all your pain. It is not easy, but it helps a little. If things go wrong, smile and rest if you must, but do not quit!

Rouge
Italy

I am thirty-five years old, and until two years ago, I thought I was only suffering from Raynaud's phenomenon. Then, after the development of small ulcers on my fingers, I had immunological tests that confirmed the diagnosis of limited scleroderma. At the moment, I have lost a bit of the elasticity of my fingers and I have some wrinkles around my mouth.

I am taking several medications. I am also under the care of a homeopath, who is giving me remedies to detoxify myself, and who has also sent me to the dentist to have my mercury fillings removed from my teeth because this could worsen the disease. I am also following a diet; I eat only whole wheat bread or pasta. I think that we can improve our condition a lot by making use of both traditional and alternative medicine.

Sharon Joy Egberts
Victoria, Australia

Six years ago, I noticed a lump in my mouth that was slowly getting bigger. Three years later, I had surgery to remove a lump on my parotid gland. It turned out to be mucosa-associated lymphatic tissue lymphoma (MALToma).

Subsequent blood tests revealed positive antinuclear antibodies (ANA). I had a CT scan, which revealed several lymph glands of pathological size. I was sent to an oncologist. I decided against treatments as radiation could cause tooth loss on the treated side, and chemotherapy could cause other problems in the future. My surgeon was sure he had gotten it all, so I decided to wait and see. I had a colonoscopy and a gastroscopy, which were both okay.

I have a checkup every six months and so far, so good. Then I went to a rheumatologist. Eventually, he diagnosed Raynaud's phenomenon and Sjögren's and told me to come back when I had any symptoms. With a chronic, incurable autoimmune disease, there was nothing he could do until I became worse. I did not like him and did not go back. I was devastated; I had a disease I could not even spell and which I had never even heard of.

My girlfriend is a nurse and my greatest support. We hit the medical library at the university and got a lot of information. Meanwhile, my mouth was getting drier. I cannot swallow a mouthful of food without a mouthful of water, or I choke. If I try to talk without sipping water, my tongue sticks to my teeth and the roof of my mouth. Bottled water has become my closest friend; I do not go anywhere without it.

I have dental phobia, so the hardest thing for me is going to the dentist three times a year, but I do anyway (thank goodness for 'happy gas!'). My teeth are full of fillings. I use a fluoride gel and clean my teeth twice a day with a special toothpaste for dry mouth.

My nose dried up, as did my vagina and my tears. I started getting dry eyes and I have trouble focusing, even with my glasses. I now use eye drops four to six times a day and see an ophthalmologist regularly.

My handbag is a portable medicine cabinet filled with lotions, potions, gels, sprays, drops, and moisturizers. I use only a very mild soap now, and I cover my body in moisturizer after showering each day.

About six months ago, I started to feel very fatigued and needed to sleep in the afternoon. My arms and legs had a dull ache. I noticed small red spots appearing on my fingers, so I requested an appointment with another rheumatologist, one who was more compassionate. She is wonderful!

When I saw her for the first time, she ordered extensive blood tests. The results showed limited scleroderma and four of the five symptoms of CREST. My ANA count has doubled. I also have elevated blood pressure, and I am a longtime sufferer of irritable bowel syndrome (IBS).

Day by day, I discover another food I cannot eat due to heartburn caused by esophageal dysfunction (the E in CREST), and my mouth and tongue burn. I cannot eat any fruit, with the exception of melons, nor can I drink fruit juices. I cannot tolerate anything spicy or acidic.

In April 2001, I had a gastroscopy, as the heartburn was getting worse. The procedure revealed that I have Barrett's esophagus with two ulcers. I was started on heartburn medication, and after more than five years of dreadful heartburn, within a week I was pain free. Within a month, I was able to eat bananas and tomatoes, and drink the odd glass of red wine again. And I was sleeping much better. Every six months, the gastroscopy is repeated.

In May, I had an attack of terrible chest pain, so I had an ultrasound, which revealed a large gallstone. The following week I had my gallbladder removed. During the next three weeks post-op, I had niggling pain and discomfort. Then one morning I woke up in agony with pain like I have never experienced in my life. I was taken by ambulance to intensive care, where subsequent tests revealed I had either a small stone in the bile duct or bile duct spasms.

The next day I had an endoscopic retrograde cholangiopancreatography procedure (ERCP) with sphincterotomy. Within twenty-four hours of the procedure, the pain increased rapidly. I was diagnosed with acute pancreatitis, a complication of the ERCP. I spent ten days in the hospital on opiate pain medication, and it took a month for my liver function tests to return to normal. I made a complete recovery and regained the six kilos I had lost!

As a routine test prior to my six-month checkup with my rheumatologist, I had an echocardiogram and a lung function test. Unfortunately, it revealed that I now have secondary pulmonary hypertension (PH). I just do not know how much more I can handle. I have read a bit about it and have an appointment in three weeks with a cardiologist who specializes in PH.

Apparently, scleroderma has shrunken the vessels between my heart and lungs. My heart has to work much harder to get the blood across to my lungs. I had been short of breath and very tired, as if someone was sitting on my chest.

On the upside, I have had no signs of return of the MALToma. I have had twelve monthly visits with the oncologist and she is happy, so I am happy.

My eyes have not gotten any drier over the past two years. My teeth are falling apart, so I still go to my dentist regularly. Soon I will be faced with having all my teeth out. I really hate the dentist, so this is a big worry for me.

In the meantime, I enjoy painting and going to art classes. I paint Australian landscapes, wild flowers, and little Aussie critters! I paint on anything I can find. It is a great source of relaxation therapy.

Update – May 2002

Nine weeks ago I was coughing and noticed a bulge just above my navel. I contacted my doctor and he sent me for an ultrasound. I was diagnosed with a large umbilical hernia. I needed that like I needed a hole in the head! He believes it was caused by the laparoscopic surgery I had twelve months ago to remove my gallbladder, as the procedure had probably weakened the abdominal wall.

Within the week I had open abdominal mesh repair surgery. Here we go again. I have had just about enough of hospitals and doctors. I spent six days in the hospital, and because of my other health problems, I take a lot longer to heal. It has been a painful, slow recovery, but I am happy to say now, eight weeks later, I am just about back to doing what I was able to do before surgery. I still have a few burning pains the doctor said could last for up to three months. I get very tired, but manage okay with an afternoon nap and early nights.

Last week, I had another test for the pulmonary hypertension. I was pleased to find out that it has progressed only marginally.

I decided to go along to a beginner's Tai Chi class. Once I learn the moves I think I will benefit from it greatly. My first class was very relaxing.

I am very lucky to have a wonderful husband of twenty-eight years and a supportive network of family and friends. I do not know what the future holds for all of us with autoimmune diseases. Hopefully, one day a cure will be found. Until then, my motto is: "When the going gets tough, the tough eat chocolate."

◆ ❖ ◆

Shirley Wright
Alabama, USA

I live in Alabama with my husband, Richard. I have two grown sons, Gregory and Christopher. I thought it was time for me to tell all about my life since I was diagnosed with limited scleroderma in 1981 at the University of Alabama, Birmingham.

When I first got sick, my symptoms were carpal tunnel syndrome. I had numbness in my right hand that was especially bothersome at night. I could not go to sleep because my hand felt dead. I would get up at night and walk the floor shaking my hand to try to get the feeling back in it. Eventually I had carpal tunnel surgery on my right wrist and it helped a lot.

After that, my hands starting turning blue and would really hurt. I will never forget the first time I knew there was something terribly wrong with me. I was in our garage, pulling down the door in the wintertime, and I completely lost all feeling in my hands. When feeling did return, it was extremely painful. I went from doctor to doctor trying to find out what was wrong with me until I was diagnosed with Raynaud's phenomenon. I had just the Raynaud's phenomenon for about three years with no other symptoms.

One year my husband caught a virus that was going around and, naturally, I caught it too, but he got better and I did not. It was as though the virus symptoms finally went away, but other symptoms took their place. I started having severe muscle weakness; it felt as though someone had attached a vacuum cleaner hose to my big toe and literally sucked all of the strength from my body. Someone who has scleroderma would understand this feeling.

One of the saddest things about this disease was that nobody understood what I was going through. I felt so alone. I went through the hardest years with scleroderma with no one to talk to about how I really felt. When my son Chris got a new computer, he gave me his old one. The computer literally changed my life for the better. I have learned that many people have scleroderma. I am not alone anymore.

I had the extreme muscle weakness for three very long years. I did not think I was ever going to feel good again. Even though my muscle strength was down to about zero, the doctors never put me on anything. I never took any of the antirheumatic drugs. They told me that sometimes it is better to wait and see just how bad the disease may progress because the medication side effects could be really bad. I truly feel that my health was overlooked a lot during this period.

They did give me medicine for the joint pain. It caused problems with my esophagus and stomach, so I stopped taking it. Mainly, I took pain relievers only if my pain was severe. When I started to have problems with my esophagus, it began with severe heartburn—like a lit match—from my throat down to my stomach. I was given medicine for that. I was bothered for years with heartburn until I started to sleep in my recliner in a slanted position. I no longer have to take medication for heartburn. I never lay down flat because if I do, I get acid reflux. I guess you can say I have learned what to do and what not to do with this disease.

Next to the muscle weakness, finger ulcers were and still are my worst problem. I know, beyond a shadow of a doubt, this is the worst pain in this world. It breaks my heart in two that anyone should ever know this pain. I have to be very careful with my hands, especially in the winter months. I stay inside nearly all the time in the winter, and when I do go out, I wear very warm gloves (preferably mittens).

I have never been able to take any of the medicine prescribed for my circulation. They give you mostly high blood pressure medicines for it, and I already have low blood pressure. For that reason, it takes me months to heal an ulcer. It is extremely important to keep an ulcer clean to avoid infection. I use tea tree oil, and cover it with tubular gauze for fingers, which I purchase at a local medical supply store.

All of this gets very depressing so my doctor put me on an anti-depressant, which has helped me very much. I have had to learn on my own how to take care of my fingers because one doctor would tell me one thing and another would tell me something totally different, so I basically had to learn what helps me and what does not. I also have learned a lot from belonging to different email message lists on the Internet. I consider all of my online friends to be my second family.

The main thing I am having problems with right now is calcium deposits right beneath the skin that will, eventually, come through the skin and cause infections. I have them on my elbows, knees, fingers, and lower arms. I have had many infections caused by the calcium deposits coming through the skin so I have had to take many antibiotics that, in turn, have caused yeast-related problems. I cannot win for losing! Ha! Not funny, but we have to laugh sometimes! I have had many calcium deposits removed from my knees and my elbows, too. When I get rid of the deposits, my problem of infection goes away.

I would like to say that despite this disease, I have managed to go on with my life. I do a few things a little differently, and there are things I can no longer do—I have to accept that. I have to or else it would get the best of me, and I do not intend to let that happen! I have to be strong when I feel I cannot be, and take life one day at a time. Nobody knows what tomorrow holds.

I find it helpful to carefully weigh everything I hear about these diseases and to care for myself in every way possible. It has helped me to be very conscious of what I eat, to stay out of stressful situations, and to exercise as much as my body will safely allow. I discuss everything with my doctor and get his opinion, however, I do not depend totally on him for every single thing, because he may not tell me absolutely everything I need to know.

I am a partner with my doctor in my care, and I should read everything I can about the disease. I keep in mind that they usually write about the worst cases. I will never forget the first time I went to the library to read about scleroderma. I was scared half to death! So I remember that it does not affect everyone the same way! Worrying about health will only make me worse because stress does affect disease.

I find hobbies are great for taking my mind off my health problems. My hobby is stained glass. I enjoy it so much, however, I must be extremely careful with my hands by wearing gloves to avoid cuts. It is probably the worst hobby a person with scleroderma could ever have! Call me stubborn. I am very proud of the work I have managed to do, despite the shape my hands are in.

Last, but not least, I laugh as much as possible, because laughter is the best medicine! I have had this disease for over twenty years and I plan on being around a lot longer! My favorite saying is: "When life gives you lemons, make lemonade!" My hope is that one day soon, they will find the cure for these diseases. Let us all work together to educate people about all of the connective tissue diseases!

◆ ❖ ◆

Susan Andrews
California, USA

Scleroderma? Me? It sounded like an exotic Italian food. I imagined being in an Italian restaurant and the waiter asking me, "Will you want breadsticks with that sclero primavera?" But I was not in an Italian restaurant; as far as I know, there is no such thing as sclero primavera. My rheumatologist was not saying "scleroderma" and ordering lab tests to determine how far this disease had progressed in my body.

Thinking back, remembering how the different symptoms appeared and not realizing that perhaps they all could be related to each other, I guess I may have had scleroderma for the last year and a half to two years and did not know it.

It probably all started in the latter part of the year 2000. I am a pharmacy technician and after over twenty-three years (at that time) of doing the same repetitive motions of typing prescriptions, making change at the cash register and the like, my wrists were beginning to give me problems. I went to my primary care physician (PCP). She thought perhaps I had carpal tunnel syndrome, the occupational hazard of repetitive motion. I was told to buy wrist braces to wear at work, which I did for about a month. Besides making me clumsy, my employer told me not to wear them as they interfered with my work performance. So I worked and am still working without them.

As I remember, time passed with little changes. Occasionally, my fingers would stiffen, become numb, or both. Within a few minutes, they would return to normal. I always thought it was the carpal tunnel syndrome flaring up. In March or April of 2001, I noticed some changes in my face. It began to feel tight, but not all the time. It also would go away, like the stiffness and numbness in my fingers. I also noticed a couple of hard spots in the jaw area on each side. Silly me, I thought it was just due to aging as I am in my late forties. My face did not bother me as far as discomfort was concerned, at least not at that time. So I did not really think much of it.

In June or July, while I was at my PCP's office for a routine visit, I mentioned the condition of my face. By that time, the hard spots had grown to include both of my cheeks. The doctor felt and examined my face, then wrote out an order for the first of many lab tests to find out what was wrong. There was no mention of scleroderma.

August and September consisted of lab tests that showed nothing. At one point, my PCP thought it might be my thyroid. It was not. Another lab test was ordered in mid-September: something different from the others for what the doctor called a "long shot." This was when the word scleroderma was first used. Those tests also came back negative and scleroderma was ruled out.

September was not over when my face suddenly flared up. The skin became very tight and pulled with every movement. At times, the discomfort was unbearable, and I could actually feel it spread down the sides of my neck and up to my temples. I was on the phone with my PCP and her staff almost every day for about two weeks relaying the symptoms. My condition was still a mystery and out of desperation, my PCP referred me to an endocrinologist. After a couple of weeks of waiting, my health insurance denied the referral with a reason that, still to this day, makes my PCP's staff laugh when mentioned. The insurance company suggested that I go see a gynecologist!

My PCP tried to help me by prescribing pain pills. One brand literally knocked me out; just one tablet before bed kept me drugged all the next day, which I did not like. Another brand worked better and caused less drowsiness, so I take it when I am at home on my day off work. Over-the-counter pain relievers had little effect on my discomfort taken singly, but my PCP's nurse suggested combining several of them, which helps me for work because they don't make me sleepy.

October brought another lab test and I noticed reflux problems during the night while trying to sleep. It became so bad that in the morning, I had the sensation of something stuck in my throat. Over-the-counter medications did not help much, so I asked my primary care physician for a prescription for heartburn medication, which seems to have solved the problem.

Along with the reflux, I noticed my hands were swelling and stiffening more, and staying that way. The ability to grasp things like coins and pieces of paper was diminishing. I could no longer pop open a soda can without using something to pry the tab up for pulling. I still thought that it was due to carpal tunnel syndrome.

Yet another lab test took place in November and my PCP submitted to my health insurance a referral to a rheumatologist. She honestly was at wits' end with the obvious conditions ruled out by all the lab tests. After all, the tests proved it was not my thyroid, or scleroderma, or any other disease. So why did I have all these weird symptoms?

In mid-November, my health insurance approved the referral. The earliest appointment I could get was over two months away in January of 2002. Surprisingly, there were no lab tests in December. By then, I had learned to deal with the facial discomfort, as well as the stiffness and swelling in my hands. It did no good to complain; it did not make any of the symptoms decrease or go away. So I dealt with them as best I could. I am still dealing with them. As my appointment grew closer, I became more anxious. What was this rheumatologist going to find? What was actually wrong with me? Was it just my imagination? I began to doubt myself. I did not want the rheumatologist to think I was a hypochondriac. Yet, I really needed to know what was going on with my face and hands.

I did not sleep well the night before the appointment. My imagination was racing through all sorts of images and by morning, I was still tired. I arrived thirty minutes early to fill out background paperwork that had been mailed in error to another "Susan Andrews" in another city. By the time I finished, forty-five minutes had passed. I turned it in to the receptionist and waited for the doctor to see me.

About five to ten minutes later, the rheumatologist called me into his office. We discussed all the paperwork I had filled out. He questioned me on some of my written answers and took notes on everything I said. After ten minutes, he directed me to an examination room. I will always remember this room as the pretzel room because this is where he examined me to see what movements I could and could not make. I was gently twisted and turned into different positions. I felt rather like a contortionist at the end of the session.

He took out what looked like a jeweler's loupe to examine my hands. He seemed most interested in the tips of my fingers. He checked my feet. He measured how much I could open my mouth, as the tight skin had affected my mouth and jaw. Throughout the examination he took notes. He asked where on my body I was sore or stiff. The entire examination took maybe fifteen minutes. Afterward, we went back into his office to discuss what he had found.

According to the rheumatologist, everything pointed to scleroderma: the tight, hard feel of my face; the stiff, swollen hands; the stiff neck I had been experiencing for the last two weeks; the tenderness of what he called ulcers on the tips of my fingers; the dryness of my hands I thought was due to the cold winter weather; and reflux (scleroderma had affected my esophagus). In other words, he deduced systemic, limited scleroderma.

He gave me a pamphlet put out by the Arthritis Foundation entitled "Scleroderma." He also gave me some samples of a fairly new drug for the reflux and asked if I needed any prednisone (steroids) for the pain and swelling. I declined that offer as I wanted to last as long as possible without having to depend on steroids. Steroids always seem to make me blow up, especially one to two weeks after finishing a course. I did not want to deal with that. He wanted to see me again in March. I sat there with a strange feeling; I was literally numb inside. It was a sensation I hope never to repeat. I had been told I did not have scleroderma. Now I do.

I was sent for more blood tests. The rheumatologist's handwriting was hard to read, but one test looked like it involved either RNA or antinuclear antibodies (ANA). As of this writing, I am still waiting to hear the results and probably will not hear until I am seen again in March.

The following week I visited my PCP. We discussed my visit with the rheumatologist. She told me she really secretly suspected I had scleroderma, even though the tests she had done were negative. She also mentioned there might be changes in some of my medications for high blood pressure, heart rate, high cholesterol, thyroid, and high blood sugar. I am a borderline Type II diabetic. Yes, I have all these ailments. I was sent for more lab tests to check my cholesterol, thyroid, and blood sugar levels. She wanted to see me in February. I will find out those results then.

So let us see: First, I am told I have scleroderma. Then, I am told I do not have scleroderma. Then I am told I do have scleroderma. Talk about swinging on a pendulum! Of course, the mental highs and lows have been hard to deal with at times. Every week or two, there is a new ache or symptom. Most recently, some of my fingers turn blue for no apparent reason and for about a minute. Then they return to normal. My shoulders and right shoulder blade ache most of the time, and the back of my neck is stiff all the time. Despite these things, I am still following my normal routines and duties the best I can.

I have always had a rather unique sense of humor. This has helped and will continue to help me get through this. I figure I will not have to worry about face lifts, but if a cure is ever found and my face returns to normal, I may find that my sagging face is dragging behind me from as far away as two thousand miles in St. Louis, Missouri! How do I feel about the other symptoms? Well, I guess it could be worse. I can think of worse diseases than scleroderma. But I was not stricken with any of those. Perhaps I am somewhat still in shock. It is funny, but I never thought I would ever get something like cancer or, until recently, some unknown disease called scleroderma. Or was that sclero primavera with breadsticks?

◆❖◆

Teresa Janey
Florida, USA

I was just diagnosed a few hours ago. Tears are streaming down my face and I am wondering what effect they will have on my dry skin. I am writing this story to scream for help. I do not even know how to feel right now. As I read the other stories, I find strength and hope, but only for the writers, not for myself.

I have not felt quite right for a few years. First, I was diagnosed with Raynaud's phenomenon. They told me to stay warm. No big deal. When the ulcer grew on my middle finger, my doctor was amazed. He had never seen anything like that before. On my follow-up visit, he told me to stay warm. No big deal.

When my heart and chest started to act crazy, I decided to surf the Internet for answers. When I found this website, all of my symptoms had names and faces. Oddly enough, they belonged together. Although my entire medical history was explained there, I thought surely I must be wrong. My brother teased me about my Internet diagnosis. Even though something was not quite right, I could not have this terrible disease.

Today, I saw a doctor who was familiar with Raynaud's phenomenon and scleroderma. Yesterday, I had insurance, but today I have to go on Medicaid because I have a life-threatening disease. And I am mad! The most ridiculous thing about this is that I am angry because I am going to get ugly and old and because I do not have the money to be sick. I have not even begun to deal with the rest of it.

Obviously, I do not yet know the proper terminology for any of these symptoms. I guess time will take care of that. Please pray for me and I will pray for all of you.

◆ ❖ ◆

Terry Krawitz
Texas, USA

A doctor who saw me in a Workers' Compensation case told me I have CREST. He spent three hours with me and was also allowed to visit my workplace. He said that the chemicals I was exposed to caused my disease, as well as the disease of several other coworkers.

I came to know this after nineteen years of working at Texas Instruments in Sherman, Texas. There have been a few of us who have been helped, but others have not been helped. For most of us, it has taken nearly fifteen years to notice something was wrong. Others have gone after the chemical company and settled out of court. Many others who really need the financial help have not had any assistance. Although Workers' Compensation has been helpful, we spend most of our time fighting them to pay the medical bills.

I have three grown children, three grandchildren, and another grandchild on the way. I am in my early fifties and it makes me nuts that I cannot work. I do a lot of ministry work to help stay busy and it helps with my pain management. I have severe neuropathy. I have learned to live with it, though it has its moments. I seem to be doing well with it. Many doctors are totally amazed at how well I am doing.

I am a very positive person now, but I was not when I first got sick. It took a long time to be diagnosed, so I tell everyone to be patient. Sometimes we fall into what is termed undifferentiated connective tissue disease (UCTD). There are Internet resources with great information, and perhaps a lot of this information can be shared with your doctors as well.

I am on oxygen most of the time. I used to be unable to walk, but I can now. I have some internal organ problems, but am managing. Breathing can be a chore at times, but then it is okay at other times. I have a cough that I have not been able to get rid of since this past fall. I have been on steroids, and I have arthritis in my spine and most of my larger joints. I have been getting injections to help with pain. I hate the weather changes as they affect me a lot, especially in the fall and spring.

I have had my fair share of depression, and most likely still have it from time to time. There are days I cannot move about and just stay in bed for the day. I have found swimming to be of great help for my fibromyalgia. It really helps when the water is warm, too.

What I can say is this: with a positive mind and good thoughts, I am able to get through the days. When things cannot get any worse, a sense of humor is a big plus. Reading or watching things with humor and laughter helps more than I can ever say.

Having a support team available is a great plus. Sharing helps with the anxiety or fears that we normally have.

I encourage everyone to find something they can do and stay with it. Look for the joy of living in the simple things of life, such as friendships.

I love to give encouragement because that is why we are here, to help everyone along this path of illness and life itself. Thank you for allowing me to share my life with you.

CHAPTER 4

In Remembrance

Frankie was my life, whom I love and will never forget,
but he gave me strength to continue and if I can help someone like you
and give you strength to go on with life, then I know he's smiling on me.
— Star, Widow of Scleroderma Patient

The Value of Support
by Judith R. Thompson

What is support? Support comes in many forms and with many faces. In many venues it means to give money; to carry; to promote the interests or cause of; to argue or vote for; to assist or help; to keep something going; or to comfort.

Since September 11, 2001, we hear the word support more than ever and rightly so. In the world of the chronically ill, we don't often hear it enough. But both patients and caregivers truly know what support means. Having someone that really understands and cares about what you are going through, especially when you need someone the most, is possibly the most important factor in the life of a chronically ill person. Be it emotional, medical, physical, financial, community or family support, or the support from a virtual stranger suffering in the same way, support is critical to someone who is ill. Without some means of support, a very ill person, more often than not, will quickly succumb to the disease process, with added depression, negative attitude or loneliness, and often a quicker end of life.

My first introduction to the value of support came shortly after my diagnosis of CREST/systemic sclerosis in 1991. The loss of independence and replacing a decent paycheck with disability income, while in a state of shock, soon followed. Even though I had family around me, no one could comprehend what I was going through. I desperately needed someone with whom I could talk. I decided to start a support group in my hometown by putting an ad in the local newspaper. I received one response. Julie Thibault called my number. She introduced herself with such relief and passion at finally finding another scleroderma person. We bonded immediately. Within the two-hour phone conversation, we had become best friends. We were scleroderma soul sisters. What an awesome feeling. We agreed to meet in person the very next day.

Our first words to each other were, "You don't look sick." Then we laughed and compared body parts, symptoms, medications, backgrounds and the diagnostic process. We discussed our concerns, depression, and past life events and found so many similarities. A favorite topic was the length of time it took to get diagnosed and all the different good and bad doctors we had come in contact with through the process. In a period of twenty-four hours, we knew each other better than anyone else we had ever met in the past forty years! It was a life-defining moment, to say the least.

We had daily contact, mostly by phone, for the next eight months. In those eight months, I never felt alone or depressed or sorry for myself. I think I even started to feel better and not as ill. I had someone in my life who knew exactly what I was experiencing and she liked me in spite of it all. We could comfortably whine and complain, joke or cry without being judged or pitied. We felt perfectly normal.

I say this because so many friends and family members turned away from me. Although I understand the fear and helplessness that others may feel when finding out that a loved one is seriously ill, I'll never understand the disappearing act that often follows. I didn't allow myself to dwell too long with these disappointments as life had suddenly become more precious and with a five- to seven-year prognosis over my head, I knew I had things I wanted and needed to do. I got busy with the business of living.

In the interim, Julie and her husband, Joe, had decided to move to Idaho. At first, I was crestfallen (pardon the pun). "Why Idaho?" I wondered. It was so far from New Hampshire. At the same time I wanted Julie to be happy and envied the adventure she was about to go on. We promised to keep in touch with letters, cards and phone calls and, eventually, both of us bought computers and had email. What a glorious thing email is! We were still as close as ever.

About a year and a half after Julie had moved to Idaho, my daughter and I went on a cross-country camping trip. This was on my list of things to do before I died. For six weeks we traveled with a visit to Julie on the itinerary. The visit was one of the highlights of the trip. By then Julie was on oxygen twenty-four/seven. Her diffuse scleroderma was progressing very quickly. At least fifty percent of her body was hardened and most of her internal organs were compromised. My disease, on the other hand, seemed to level off and I was feeling pretty good.

Soon after my trip was over, Julie was admitted to the hospice program, as her doctor gave her six months to live. This was 1995. I was beside myself as I had just seen her and, except for having to drag around the oxygen tank, she seemed so full of energy, had a happy attitude, and was busy in her husband's and her new metal art design company. Even when ill, life can be busy, exciting, fruitful and "normal," if one has a good, positive mind-set. Julie had a zest for life and fought the doctors and insurance companies every step of the way. She never took no for an answer if the opportunity to try a promising new treatment presented itself. She used her determination to live, to seek out the best doctors. She was one of the most assertive patients I had ever seen. She even managed to get out of the hospice program, and she stayed out for four more years!

On September 16, 1999, I received an email from Julie.

"Been feeling poorly. Mostly weak and not wanting to do anything. So very glad to get your card and know I have email. Had mom and dad here for a week visit. Was okay. They left this A.M. I have so much work to do and no energy to do any of it. I just don't know what to do. I rest, but it doesn't help at all; still very tired. In fact, I'm too tired now, but wanted to get something off to you ASAP. Will write when I have more energy. Sorry, Julie"

The very next day, I received another email.

"Just found out today, I have approximately six months. The cancer markers I had done last week showed activity in the cancer spread. Been in shock all day. In and out of tears. Start chemo pump on Tuesday and CAT scans on Wednesday, just to see what's growing. I hate CAT scans. May go into hospice again. The lady I like is out of town until next week. So lots will happen next week. Been feeling very tired. So very much work to do with the company, and of course the house stuff, too. I just can't get the motivation or drive to get any work done. Too much to handle right now. So happy you love email and net. Mind boggling to know how much info is just out there. Going to take a bath now, may make me feel better. Email you later kiddo. Luv ya, Jules"

I called her immediately. She always asked how I was feeling first. I ignored the question, as I felt guilty for feeling so good. She assured me that she had everything she needed and that her husband, Joe, was taking good care of her.

On Thanksgiving, November 28, I received this email from Julie.

"Today is the day to give thanks for all the people who love you. So today, I must give thanks to my best friend, Judy, who is the best friend on earth. No human could ask for a better friend. I'm so glad we are friends. I go for yet another CAT scan Thursday, December 2, to see what's in my stomach. I have gained so much weight, now at 162 pounds. My stomach is so big the doctor asked if I could be pregnant. I look six to nine months along. Very uncomfortable. One good thing, my hair is growing back. Yea! I'm glad it's on the move. Gotta keep this short, dinner is at 12:00, too early for me, oh, well. Thanks again for being my friend and all that goes along with it. Love, Julie"

I knew she was starting to say goodbye.

My daughter and I had gone through hospice volunteer training (to prepare us for my death), and I knew saying goodbye was part of the dying process. All I could think about was her hair growing back. Julie had gorgeous, natural, thick, blond hair, which had always been her pride and joy. I emailed her back and told her I felt the same and then started doing the bald hair jokes. I always turn to humor when I don't know what to say.

December came fast. I received a birthday invitation from Joe. He told me he knew it would be Julie's last birthday. He had planned a limo to a fancy restaurant. Unfortunately, I had no money for that big of a trip at that time of year. So I decided to do a birthday video. With help from my daughter, her fiancé, and my boyfriend, I wrote a skit and got props and set up the production. It was a silly, loving recap of our relationship.

In the meantime, I received another email from Julie on December 7th.

"In about one-half hour, I go to the doctor to have my lung drained. The CT scan showed fluid in the lung as well as in the tummy. Since he wouldn't get the fluid out of my tummy last week, I'm not too sure I'm thrilled about him trying to drain my lung. I have started coughing again this week and been miserable every night. I just have to do something! I sit upright and try to get some sleep, but have to get up every two or three hours to take meds. Life can really suck sometimes. Joe is going with me for a while. Just to talk to the doctor and, hopefully, while the procedure is in progress. They can blow out the lung easily, then that means a fast trip to the hospital across the street. I better take a tranquilizer now. I'm getting stressed. I'll email you when I get back and things settle down some. See ya, Julie"

Meanwhile, I was working on her birthday video. I wanted to get it out soon since her birthday was on the eighteenth. On December 16th, I received an email. Even with all that she was going through, she still always managed to think of me.

"Hi Judy, I had to buy my computer. No benefits for me. But there is an organization. I'll have to see if I can find them again and let you know. I got on Hospice Medicare today! A girl at the Cancer Center found a way to get me covered. Yea! My sister is coming tomorrow to see me. Should be a good time of shopping and eating! Love ya, Kiddo. Be on the lookout for a gift I sent your way. Julie"

The video had been sent to Joe and on the day after her birthday, I received this email.

"Judy, it has taken me what seems like days to get the courage to view your wonderful video. I knew it would be delightful as well as a tearjerker (which it was). How did I get so lucky to have a friend like you? Like the tape says, it was meant to be. Just like you

and that cutie, Dan. Thank you ever so much to take the time and effort to go over our history together. Lots of years have passed and good and sad times, too. My body keeps fighting the big fight of life. But I'm tired. So many things happen to the body. My legs are swelling to the knees now; not a good sign. The doctors just give up since they feel "you are gonna die anyway." I hate them for that attitude. We are almost ready for Christmas, some wrapping to do and, of course, the prime rib dinner at home. I want brownies, pound cake and cookies. But I must eat regular food first. Hey have you tried Senokot-S? It really works for me. Pretty expensive, but it works without pain or cramping. You ought to at least try a small bottle of it for a few days. You must get it with the "S" on the end. Means stool softener and laxative combined. Try it. Well, enjoy your time with that handsome man of yours. Love you and think of you daily, Julie"

Julie had told me in a phone call that she didn't think she would make the New Millennium. But the year 2000 celebrations came and went. Julie was still with us.

I was beginning to get more phone calls from Joe, as Julie was too tired. I could tell Joe needed the support now. I told him that he was an angel and a man to be admired and honored for the way he had supported Julie through all of this. She spent more and more time in bed. I didn't quite know how to deal with this turn of events. My five- to seven-year sentence had come and gone. I was busy figuring how to start living differently with no timeframe hanging over me as I was doing fairly well. Other than a year-long liver flare and worsening bowel problems, a couple of finger ulcers, the usual Raynaud's and vasculitis, I felt pretty good. I felt guilty that I was doing so well. I knew it was a short matter of time for Julie.

I tried to get her to talk about her feelings of death, all the while trying to assure her that there was life after death and all kinds of other spiritual mumbo jumbo. I kept telling her how important her life was and how fortunate she was to have a husband as loving and supportive as Joe. What do you say? You say everything and anything.

As Julie succumbed to the last throes of scleroderma, I began analyzing this disease again. I had become somewhat complacent and accepting as I valued being out of the rat race and was able to do the things I loved to do, such as writing, reading, needlepoint, painting, doing jigsaw puzzles, and living. My time was my time, and I relished it. Julie was still fighting. To me, she fought too hard and left herself open to some quackery and every new test and medicine that came down the pike. She did not want to die. I feel it left her more vulnerable to opportunistic infections.

She got rickets, which she told me was extremely painful, and all kinds of weird side effects from some of the procedures she went through. On February 7, 2000, I received this email.

"Hi Kiddo. Thought I would bring you up to date. I've had three lung taps to drain the right cancer-ridden lung. The doctor wants to do a pleurodesis. If all goes well, the hospital stay will be five days. It's a type of talc glue to close the holes the cancer has created. By draining the lung with a chest tube and then filling it with the slurry of talc-like substance. Creating sticky glue-like substance to adhere the outer lining of the lung to the ribs (I think). Been sick with coughing and lung infections almost constantly. Antibiotics just keep infection in check. As far as the brain tumor goes, I have terrible right leg shaking. Comes and goes, thank God. Some light-headed feeling and a few headshakes as well. But other than that it's quiet. Just hired a new woman today. She's super. Training will be a snap as she knows so much about computers and software programming. Teddy, Joe, and his mom, Eleanor, all feel the stresses of my four-month prognosis. I just accept it and go on. I've been on hospice one month now and am glad they are taking care of me. A great bunch of people. Anyways, I got your card today. Where do you find them? A store? Catalog? Internet? Hope all is well with you and Dan. Lots of love, Julie"

On February 8, I sent this email to Julie.

"Hi Julie, glad you got the Valentine's card. I think I got that one at Target. My daughter's planning her wedding. Lots going on, but it's starting to catch up. I feel like sleeping for a few days. I'll say my prayers that the new lung-plug treatment works. But you have already beaten all the odds. You could probably make it into Ripley's Believe It or Not J. I love and miss you. Give my best to Joe. So happy that you hired a girl to help. Judy"

I never heard from Julie again.

She never recuperated from the last lung treatment. Joe called me several times telling me what was happening to her. I was hearing the true caregiver's side of a disease. What he went through and did for his wife makes my friendship and support seem minuscule at best. It was awful to hear. I couldn't imagine actually living with what Joe was dealing with. Being sick was the easy side of a disease. Taking care of a sick loved one is much harder emotionally.

She never was lucid or had enough strength to even speak on the phone. On March 20, 2000, Julie died. She died in her husband's arms and fairly peacefully.

Except for Julie, I really had no support for dealing with my scleroderma. I'm sure my daughter would be there if things got bad. And I know hospice would be there, too. And once I discovered this website, I found support and a purpose to "get on with it."

Support, however it comes, is a godsend! All one can share is oneself and sharing a similar experience, be it good or bad, is worth its weight in gold.

A. M. Keyes
Surviving Daughter of Pulmonary Fibrosis/Scleroderma Patient
North Carolina, USA

My father died on February 9, 2002, from pulmonary fibrosis, a complication of the disease scleroderma.

My father was diagnosed with scleroderma twenty-two years ago. I remember well the day the doctor informed my father, mother, and me of his findings. He told us that there was no cure. A knot formed in my stomach.

It was the same knot that came back on February 9, while listening to the doctor outside of my dad's hospital room tell me that we were going to lose him. My father held on to see all of his children and grandchildren before falling into a peaceful and eternal sleep. It was a most spiritual and heartfelt transition, although we are left with a deep void.

It happened so fast, once it started, that now as I look back on it, I don't know if there was anything that could have saved him. I want to believe that the doctors did all they could.

Still, I miss him terribly and have decided that I want to become involved in making others aware of this disease. I was amazed that people knew very little about scleroderma and the many forms it can take. In memory of my dad, I would like to change that.

For all of you who have loved ones out there with the disease, hold them close and relish each and every day. I know I did and when my daddy lost his battle, I know that we gave it our all.

I believe that, in time, a cure will be found, and knowing the type of man my father was, he would want that, in spite of the fact that it could not save him. To all of you, be strong and hold onto your faith.

◆ ❖ ◆

Archie H. Bailey
Surviving Spouse of Sue Hartwick Bailey
Michigan, USA

Time has passed since Sue's death. Only those who have experienced the grieving process can understand the profound agony death presents to friends and loved ones.

Susan (Hartwick) Bailey was my wife for forty-two years. Our forty-third wedding anniversary followed her death by eleven days.

In July 1990, Sue's rheumatologist told her that her puzzling physical symptoms could be signaling the onset of one of a variety of autoimmune diseases such as lupus or scleroderma. "Only time will tell," her physician said ominously, "We'll have to wait to see what develops."

Sue's official Certificate of Death, issued in August 1999, objectively listed her immediate cause of death as cor pulmonale, which is a disease of the heart characterized by thickening and dilation of the right ventricle that was secondary to disease of the lungs and their blood vessels. Other conditions listed as contributing to her death were pulmonary hypertension and progressive systemic scleroderma.

After her death, like others, I probably had many of the classic symptoms of clinical depression including depressed mood, loss of interest or pleasure in activities, changes in sleep patterns, loss of energy, and, at times, a diminished ability to think clearly or to concentrate.

Writers from ancient times to Shakespeare to C. S. Lewis' *A Grief Observed* and Ruth Coughlin's *Grieving: A Love Story* have written hundreds of books about the grieving process from their own perspective. All are very personal and revealing and all tell a different story.

As a compulsive reader, the first place I turned for information about how to handle my loss, and perhaps find some solace, was to books. I made many trips to the local bookstore trying to read through my visual blur. I'd go directly to the section labeled "Grieving" and proceed, almost shelf-by-shelf, one book at a time, searching for a sentence, a phrase or thought that would inspire me or help me to return home and face that empty house.

Although touched by the personal stories of others and impressed by the written advice of professionals, I discovered that nothing applied to me. The grieving process is indeed an individual experience.

How it all began...talk about fate! I met Sue Hartwick through a one-line ad in the classified's help wanted section of the *Detroit News* in 1953.

Or, to be more accurate, I should say that my father discovered Sue for me. My father was always trying to find me a job. He wanted me to keep busy. The ad wasn't a matchmaker-type ad, like those that seem so popular today. It simply stated: "Wanted, canoeing instructor for summer camp in the Petoskey area. Experience required." A phone number was included.

My father was convinced that the camp director was looking for me. I contacted her and was invited for an interview by one of the most interesting and truly eccentric women I have ever met. She asked about my canoeing experience as a camper in the rugged Georgian Bay area of Ontario. During the interview, she even asked me to sing a couple of camp songs that I had learned at a camp in Canada.

The only question she didn't ask me was the most important question of all. If she had asked, "How old are you, Archie?" the interview would have ended there. If she had known that I was only sixteen years old and in the tenth grade, I would never have been hired and would never have met Sue. Even at sixteen, I must have looked older than my age. Maybe it was the early start of a lifelong receding hairline. But, I was also a former Canadian with all the appropriate social graces. I promptly stood when a woman entered the room, my manners were almost quietly British, and I still had a semi-Canadian accent. I rolled words like "aboot" and sometimes added a soft "eh" at the end of a sentence.

The camp director knew she was getting a bargain. The salary for the entire summer was one hundred dollars and on June 6, 1953, I boarded a Greyhound bus in Highland Park, Michigan, and headed for a summer-long job as a canoeing instructor on Walloon Lake, not far from Ernest Hemingway's summer home.

~~~~

In 1990, scleroderma caught both Sue and me by complete surprise. We were attending a political dinner. During the meal, I looked down and noticed that Sue's hands were deep purple from wrists to fingertips. Their appearance clearly startled me.

Sue was a popular county commissioner at the time, and we were attending a political function at a local VFW Hall in her district. It was a warm August night, but we were sitting near an air-conditioning vent. The slight, indirect cool breeze was enough to cause her hands to almost instantly turn dark purple. I remember asking, "Sue, what's wrong? Look at your hands." I touched them and they were ice cold. "What's going on here?" I asked.

"Oh, it's probably just from shaking hands with him," she said pointing to the Republican nominee for governor, who was also campaigning at the dinner. Clearly, her condition wasn't a result of shaking hands with the Republican candidate.

Her purple hands were one of the first signs of what can be the onset of progressive systemic scleroderma and several other medical conditions. It is called Raynaud's phenomenon and it is a disorder that can affect the blood vessels in the fingers, toes, ears and nose. It is characterized by episodic, vasospastic attacks that cause the blood vessels to constrict. Recent research shows that Raynaud's phenomenon may affect five to ten percent of the general population in the United States. Women are more likely than men to experience the disorder.

Sue soon learned from specialists that Raynaud's phenomenon could be symptomatic of connective tissue diseases like lupus and scleroderma. There are various treatments for Raynaud's phenomenon, but none worked for Sue. Keeping her hands warm with insulated mittens was the only remedy that worked for her.

No one ever commented directly to Sue about her mittens, but she did receive stares from people at the local supermarket when they saw her in June, July or August shopping in the frozen food department wearing her mittens. Those mittens soon became part of her year-round daily attire.

~~~~

Sue began her summer job as a counselor at Hilltop Camp the same day I started as the canoeing instructor. She had been interviewed and hired by "Madame," the title the camp director preferred, so nicknamed as a student on the campus of Michigan State College (now University). In June, Sue traveled by train from her home in Grand Rapids to Petoskey. We all arrived a few days before the campers.

On the day we first met, I was working with another counselor in the camp's Nature Cabin helping him unpack and catalogue materials. Sue came in and "Nature Boy," as the Nature Instructor was called, introduced me to her. He knew Sue. He was from Grand Rapids, too and a student at Michigan State College.

Sue was born and raised in Grand Rapids where she attended public schools and graduated from Union High School. Her father was a postal employee and her mother worked in the lamp department of a local department store. Others have expressed it in words and song, and I can't add anything new or original, other than I felt an immediate connection with this very attractive girl from Grand Rapids. I anticipated a great summer.

~~~~

At first it was difficult to understand why someone with Raynaud's phenomenon would be sent to a physician specializing in arthritis. But since scleroderma is a connective tissue disease, Sue's general practitioner referred her to an arthritis specialist for a consultation.

During that period of time, I wasn't involved in Sue's day-to-day healthcare, so she went for the consultation alone. She said to me that night, "The doctor said it could be any number of things: lupus, scleroderma, or a half a dozen other diseases, which I can't remember now." She also said, "It could just be Raynaud's and that I should try to keep my hands warm. She wants to see me in six months." Neither of us was alarmed.

~~~~

The summer of 1953 at camp on Walloon Lake was a turning point in my life. I didn't realize it at the time, but it was indeed an early rite of passage. No one at camp knew I was sixteen and I didn't volunteer the information. I tried my best to fit in. I told Sue many years later that I felt like Montgomery Clift in the classic film *A Place in the Sun*. Sue's response was, "Archie, aren't you stretching it a bit?"

The other counselors were attending a college or university somewhere. Most were in a fraternity or sorority. Sue was a Gamma Phi Beta in East Lansing. Another was a student at Harvard, a school I'd only read about. I tried to blend in with the staff in every way I could. That summer I drank my first beer, kissed my first girl, fell in love with the works of Hemingway and Upton Sinclair. I was introduced to a different world beyond the rough and tumble life of urban Highland Park.

In the middle of the summer, I somehow got up enough courage to ask Sue for a date. She accepted and we went with "Nature Boy" and his date to see a movie in Petoskey. The movie was *Shane* with Alan Ladd and Brandon DeWilde. The film impressed me. Today, I can still whistle almost the entire musical score, and I can repeat many of the main characters' famous lines.

Many years later Sue said she remembered the movie, but not much else about that night. She never liked to look back in time. I bought the videotape of the movie and whenever I played it, Sue would say, "Oh, oh, here we go—Archie's in his Shane mood again."

At the end of summer, I gave Sue my address and told her that I wanted to stay in touch. Apparently, she did, too. She went back to Michigan State and I returned as an eleventh grader at Highland Park High School.

~~~~

Sue's pictures in the family photo album, from 1990 until her death in 1999, reveal a progressive change in her appearance. I didn't really notice the change until I was going through the photo albums sorting pictures after her death.

During the early 1990s, Sue was the Chief Deputy County Clerk. There were several posed pictures showing her seated at her desk. Even through her smile, she seemed to be getting more pale with each photograph. Clearly, she didn't feel well and her appearance was slowly changing.

During this same period, she was increasingly annoyed by what she considered to be minor but persistent physical ailments. Her fingers were beginning to swell. For the first time in her life, she had trouble taking her rings off when she washed her hands or washed the dishes. Small red dots began to appear on the palms of her hands (physicians refer to this as "telangiectasia") and on her tongue and face.

She retired from public life in 1994, but continued to be active in a variety of organizations dedicated to the welfare of children. The Michigan Supreme Court appointed her to an important foster child advocacy board. At the same time, she was becoming a full-time grandmother and enjoying the role. Her condition was developing into a serious and chronic life-threatening illness, but it didn't slow her down. She complained to no one, except her physician, about her medical problems.

~~~~

In 1954, I graduated from high school and enrolled at Highland Park Junior College. Sue completed her sophomore year at Michigan State. In 1953 and 1954, we sent each other cards and notes at Christmas. In 1955, I was in Miami, Florida, for Christmas and my father forwarded my mail to me there.

One day on the steps of the main post office in Miami, I opened a Christmas card from Sue. Her return address was Royal Oak, Michigan, not far from my home in Highland Park. I remember looking at my friend and saying something to him like, "Hey, we're heading home tomorrow. Sue Hartwick lives in Royal Oak now and I want to see her!" My friend seemed somewhat relieved because all he had heard from me for the previous two years was Sue Hartwick, Sue Hartwick, and Sue Hartwick.

He thought he was finally going to meet Sue Hartwick. We left for Michigan the next day, probably making the trip in record time in my beat-up 1949 Ford. The day I arrived home, I called Sue. We started to see each other and in August 1957, we were married in Grand Rapids.

~~~~

In August 1994, Sue was at our cottage on Green Lake, near Interlochen, getting everything ready for the Labor Day weekend. Traditionally, this was Sue's favorite summer holiday. We always celebrated that final weekend of the season with good friends from Grand Rapids. She always wanted her cottage and the weekend to be just right.

I arrived early Friday afternoon and found Sue lying down on the couch in the living room trying to keep warm under a heavy blanket. The temperature outside was in the eighties. She said she had a slight headache and felt a little lightheaded. I told her not to get up and to just lie there. I told her I wanted to take a short walk down the road behind the cottage to stretch my legs. Another tradition, she wanted to go, too. We walked a short distance from the cottage and Sue said, "I've got to go back. I can't go on. I don't feel well." We turned around and inside the cottage she returned to the couch and got under the blanket. Something was definitely wrong; Sue rarely complained about anything. Later that night, our friends arrived and Sue did her best not to show her discomfort.

The next day we all went for our traditional end-of-the-summer boat ride around the lake. Sue didn't really want to go, but she wanted that weekend to be perfect. I have a picture of her on the boat in a heavy hooded sweatshirt. I took a lot of pictures that weekend. That night we went to Traverse City for dinner. At the restaurant, we all ordered a drink and our meals. Sue was very talkative—almost nonstop, about nothing. We were served our food and Sue didn't touch her dinner. She never picked up a fork. She sat there and talked nonstop. Finally, her friend Betty took her by the hand and asked, "Sue, what's wrong? Something must be wrong." With tears in her eyes, Sue answered, "Oh, Betty, I don't know. I just don't feel well." We helped her to the car and headed for the cottage.

~~~~

During 1957 to 1959, I completed my undergraduate degree at Wayne State University in Detroit while Sue moved up through the ranks of Oakland

County's Social Work Division. In later years, she reminded me from time to time when she seemed to think I was too self-confident, that the four college degrees I eventually earned would not have been possible if she had not worked for both of us those first two years. I agreed and, in fact, I told her many times that everything I achieved personally and professionally would not have been possible without her. I wasn't kidding. She was a great inspiration and motivator.

After graduation, I worked for Procter & Gamble in Saginaw. Although I was successful, I realized that it wasn't for me. I always wanted to be a teacher. So we moved to East Lansing for a year while I completed the requirements for a Master's degree and a Michigan teaching certificate. Again, Sue worked for the Ingham County Probate Court while I was in school.

In September 1961, I began teaching for the Livonia Public Schools and Sue returned to the Oakland County Probate Court. They were pleased to see her return. We moved into our first home on Ellwood Avenue in Berkley that we purchased for twelve thousand five hundred dollars, wondering how we would ever be able to pay off the mortgage.

The Berkley years were exciting for both of us. Sue and I enthusiastically entered the world of politics. The Berkley City Council recognized Sue's ability and appointed her to the Oakland County Board of Supervisors. I was elected to the Berkley Board of Education. We met friends and future leaders like Carl and Sander Levin, Jim Blanchard, and many more.

In November 1963, I chaired the annual Phil Hart Dinner—one week before President Kennedy was assassinated. Newly elected Senator Edward Kennedy was the guest speaker. Sue sat next to him with me at the head table. It was heady stuff for Sue and Archie.

~~~~

We left the Traverse City restaurant that night in August 1994, took Sue back to the cottage and put her to bed. The next day I drove her to the emergency room of a Flint hospital. We were both shocked to see the triage nurse write down and circle in red that her blood pressure was 245/120. The ER doctor said Sue had malignant hypertension. He had no idea what was causing it. "That's for your family doctor to determine," he said. It was at that moment that we began our long journey through the maze called "the practice of modern American medicine."

It was Labor Day weekend. The ER physician reviewed her status and gave her medicine that brought her blood pressure down slightly. He said,

"I'm going to send you home. I want you to see your own doctor tomorrow morning." That response didn't sound right to us, but we were new to the system. The next morning her blood pressure had gone back up.

Sue had been seeing a new general practitioner (GP). The doctor was a woman and Sue liked her. She had always wanted a woman doctor. I never knew much about that physician except that she was a woman. Sue was impressed. When Sue saw her the next day, she was given another drug to try to bring the blood pressure down to an acceptable level. If it didn't work, Sue was told to come back to the office the next morning and they would try something else. I monitored Sue's blood pressure at home, and I could clearly see that the medicine wasn't working.

We were back in the office early the next morning. The nursing staff took Sue into the examination room and in about fifteen minutes, a nurse rushed out and asked me to come with her. "There is a problem," she said, "please come quickly." Sue was lying unconscious on an examination table. Her eyes were open and widely dilated. She seemed to be staring at the ceiling. Her doctor and another physician were trying everything to help Sue regain consciousness. What they were doing wasn't working. They called for an ambulance, and we returned to the same emergency room of the local hospital; the same one where that physician had sent her home just a few days before.

~~~~

In 1967, Sue and I had been married for ten years. For some reason, we were unable to have children. Doctors at Beaumont Hospital in Royal Oak, Michigan, had given both of us a clean bill of health, but it just didn't happen. In September of that year, we adopted our first child.

Sue's mother had been living with us for the previous ten months through the final agonizing and fatal stages of colon cancer. Sue wanted to get out of the Berkley house. We both needed a change. So I took a job as a high school counselor in Grand Rapids and in September, Sue, our new baby girl and I packed up, cut our Berkley ties, and moved to Grand Rapids.

We lived in Grand Rapids for one year. What a year it was! The day I reported to school, I couldn't get in the building. The Board of Education had imposed a staff "lockout" in a labor dispute with the teachers' union. The lockout lasted about three weeks. Later in the year, the high school was rocked by racial disturbances that brought the Michigan State Police Task Force to the building. Events at the school were reported in the *New*

York Times. National Guard officers slept in the gymnasium for about two weeks until the situation settled down. At the same time, the principal was fired as a scapegoat for the disturbances. Later, his replacement was fired for stealing school funds. It was a wild year.

Sometime that year, I met the Director of Personnel of the Flushing Community Schools, and he offered me an administrative position as Director of Guidance Services with the school district. I accepted and we packed up and moved to Flushing, Michigan, after only one interesting year in Grand Rapids. It was to be our final move.

~~~~

Sue's first hospitalization made one thing very clear to both of us: the importance of the role of the primary care physician (PCP) in the treatment of scleroderma patients.

When Sue arrived at the hospital by ambulance from her doctor's office, we received a number of surprises. The first was that Sue's blood pressure was really out of control, and she was in acute kidney failure. The medication she had received the day before had lowered her blood pressure too rapidly and some of her veins had collapsed. She was taken from the emergency room to a semiprivate room where we got our second surprise. We learned that Sue's GP didn't have hospital privileges. We learned that information from a physician who came into the room and announced that he was standing in for "Dr. So-and-So," that he cared for all of "Dr. So-and-So's" patients who were hospitalized, but that "Dr. So-and-So" was out of town for the weekend. When "Dr. So-and-So" returned on Monday, "Dr. So-and-So" would be caring for her.

In the meantime, the "stand-in," as I called him, picked up Sue's chart, scanned it, and then said with some urgency to the nurse who was present, "Move Mrs. Bailey to ICU immediately. I don't like what I see on this chart. She will need full-time nursing care. Get her there as quickly as possible."

That was the most decisive action taken by anyone up to that point. I asked the doctor if he could take over and supervise Sue's case. He agreed but wanted to talk with Sue to make sure she approved. At this point, Sue was still unconscious. When he finally got a chance to ask her several days later, her response was one that none of us forgot. Meeting this doctor proved, in the long run, to be a very lucky break for Sue.

He immediately assembled a team of heart, lung, kidney, eye, blood, and neurological specialists from the local medical community. They sent blood and urine specimens to the University of Michigan for special tests. During Sue's hospital stay, her condition ranged from critical to stable. She drifted in an out of consciousness and, at times, had very limited mental acuity.

Amazingly, ten days after she had been admitted, Sue went home. She had been through a great deal during that time, much of which she didn't remember. It would be the first of many hospital stays. Sue's new doctor broke the news that, indeed, she did have scleroderma. Her blood tests didn't clearly indicate the disease. In fact, throughout the entire progress of the disease, she never passed the blood test for scleroderma, but small things, when put together, seemed to make the diagnosis positive.

~~~~

When we arrived in Flushing, we thought of the town as a small quiet suburban community nestled along the banks of the Flint River. I had read Edmund Love's book *The Situation in Flushing*, and I actually thought Flushing would be the way he described it. I soon learned that his book was indeed—as the author told me himself many years later—pure fiction.

I enjoyed my job at Flushing High School. During our first year in town, Sue was named Branch Manager of the Michigan Secretary of State Office in Flushing. The position was a political appointment made by Michigan's Secretary of State Richard Austin. The Genesee County Democratic Party and powerful UAW officials had recommended another person to Austin for the position.

Not for the first nor last time, Sue challenged both those authorities with great poise and used her contacts, established as an Oakland County official, to appeal directly to Austin. He appointed Sue and she served as Branch Manager for almost two years until the position became a state civil service position, and the office was closed. In the process, Sue ran the office with efficiency and met hundreds of Flushing-area residents, and they liked her.

In 1971, we adopted our second daughter. Soon, Sue was appointed by the City Council to the Flushing Planning Commission and, eventually, ran unopposed for the Flushing City Council. This was the beginning of a winning streak of elections for her that lasted until she became Chief Deputy County Clerk in 1981. During her entire career as an elected official, she never lost an election. People liked Sue Bailey.

Sue's first hospitalization made both of us realize that our lives were changed forever. We began to do what every person diagnosed with scleroderma should do; we tried to learn as much about the disease as possible. Almost everyone's response to the word "scleroderma" is "sclera-what?" We soon discovered that the only people who knew anything about scleroderma were people whose own lives or loved ones had been affected by the disease.

There are only a few scleroderma specialists in Michigan. One is located at Hutzel Hospital in Detroit. After Sue got home from the hospital and was rested and somewhat refreshed, we visited the specialist in Detroit.

We described what had happened to Sue in the hospital in Flint and shared all of Sue's test results and other records: acute kidney failure; malignant hypertension; an insidious swelling of her fingers; a thickening of skin on both hands; some difficulty breathing; red spots on her face and hands, along with many other related problems.

The doctor said that all these conditions, especially kidney failure, were characteristic of scleroderma. The specialist's next comment was, indeed, ominous. She said that scleroderma varies in severity and progression. She told us that some scleroderma patients live with symptoms for many years, while others can have rapidly progressive and fatal heart, lung, and kidney involvement. The course of the disease, she said, is both variable and unpredictable. She said that future medical care would, basically, be the management of Sue's symptoms.

Subsequently, we saw a second specialist at the University of Michigan Medical Center. He provided the same prognosis. "Much research is currently underway in dealing with scleroderma and searching for the cause and a cure," he said. "In the meantime, we can only treat the symptoms."

By this time, Sue was feeling better physically and she determined that "sclera-whatever" was not going to slow her down. Those who knew Sue best—her friends—will testify that until and near the very end, Sue tried hard to maintain a normal life. Slowing down wasn't her style. She was now a full-time grandmother and she put all her energy into that role and into a few committees on which she served. She chose her projects carefully.

~~~~

In 1980, Sue filed to run in the Democratic primary as a candidate for County Commissioner. She was going to take on the incumbent. At first, she was a reluctant candidate. A friend and political advisor helped me to convince Sue that she could win. In the past, I had been the candidate several times while Sue worked on the campaigns. This time our roles were reversed, and I was on the sidelines planning, raising money, researching issues, and putting up signs while Sue did the vote-seeking.

Sue was a very effective campaigner. She capitalized on her personality and people-skills and the fact that she was a woman out to claim some political ground. She campaigned door-to-door that entire summer. She walked in parades and shook hands at a variety of political events. She even rode a mule in a local parade. Campaigning was exhausting and many of her friends pitched in to help. There were days when I would come home from work at the end of the day to find Sue asleep on the couch with campaign brochures still clutched in her hand. After dinner, she would hit the trail with friends knocking on doors until it got too dark to continue.

The political pundits and local papers said there was no way she could win. The incumbent was too powerfully entrenched. They said Sue didn't have enough experience.

It was even hinted that it was somewhat presumptuous of her to run. The large metropolitan paper strongly endorsed her opponent and lauded him for his experience. On Election Day, she worked the polls from 8 A.M. to 8 P.M. nonstop. She had given the campaign everything she had. It paid off big. She buried the incumbent everywhere, even in his own part of the county.

Sue's opponent in the general election was a highly respected businessman from her own community. Again, the largest local newspaper endorsed her opponent. Once again, her goal was to knock on every door in the district. On Election Day in November, she won again.

In January, she began a partisan political career that would span a decade. She would run in ten more campaigns for County Commissioner and never come close to losing any one of them. At the same time, she began to emerge as a leader in county government at the state level.

~~~~

On her first office visit to her new PCP (the "stand-in") after her hospitalization, he smiled and asked, "Is this the same Sue Bailey I saw in the hospital last week? It can't be!" Of course, Sue had worked hard to look good. She was determined not to allow her illness to alter her life outwardly in any visible way. That was to be her approach for the next four years—the last four years of her life.

Sue was tough. Even though her health forced her to sever many public responsibilities, she knew her three grandchildren were counting on her to continue to be a wonderful, caring grandmother—or "Mema," as they called her. Circumstances were such that she was required to become an almost full-time grandmother, active in the daily care of her grandchildren. Her doctor told me many times during the coming months, "Archie, you must keep Sue stress-free as much as possible. Stress is the worst thing for her at this time. Scleroderma is progressive and episodes can be triggered by stress." Frequently, as a modern mother and grandmother, avoiding stress just wasn't possible.

In 1998, our oldest grandson, who was eight at the time, stumbled, then fell and had trouble getting up while playing soccer. Throughout the week, he complained of pain in his leg and then fell again the following Saturday. I took him to a local doctor who X rayed his leg and hip and then told me he had Perthes disease. The disease involves the disintegration of the hip and leg bone where they join together. The doctor said to me that day, "This is very serious. Something like this requires the very best specialist available. In this case, she is at the University of Michigan Medical Center. I'll call and make an appointment for you to see her as soon as possible."

After several diagnostic visits to the University of Michigan Medical Center, our grandson had major surgery and was placed in a cast from armpits to toes. His legs were held apart with a wooden pole from knee to knee. Circumstances at the time required that he stay with Sue and me to recuperate. We pulled out the hide-a-bed in the family room and for eight weeks, despite her rapidly declining health, we cared for the little guy around the clock. In many ways, it was a pleasure for us to have him at our house. Caring for him helped Sue focus on something other than her own medical problems. Believe it or not, the three of us—grandmother, grandfather, and patient—had plenty of laughs and good times as his hip healed. His brother, Bradley, and sister, Erica, provided lots of good times also.

It was shortly after our grandson's full recovery that tests on Sue's lungs showed evidence of increasingly low diffusion rates. No one told us, but we both knew that scleroderma was attacking her heart, lungs, and kidneys simultaneously. *The Merck Manual* states that: "Scleroderma patients' prognosis is poor if cardiac, pulmonary, or renal manifestations are present early."

From this point in time until six months before her death, Sue did her best to face the challenges presented by her disease. For example, she remained active on the board of directors of various groups dedicated to the welfare of children. The Michigan Supreme Court had appointed Sue to the Foster Care Review Board, and it was the last board from which she would resign because of her health. During this period, I drove Sue to her meetings and helped her to the meeting rooms since she could only walk short distances unassisted.

She never gave up. During this same period, she planned the wedding of our oldest daughter. She did her best to live up to her reputation as an effective organizer. Of course, the wedding was a success. Everything was perfect. Looking now at those wedding pictures, it was obvious that she continued to look pale and drawn.

With a disease such as scleroderma where there is no known cause and no cure, the PCP can only do what the specialist had told us would be necessary: treat the symptoms. Distressing symptoms now began to rapidly develop into major medical crises.

Initially, her kidneys caused the most trouble. Her renal specialist decided, in consultation with others, that she needed to begin dialysis. Since her veins were too fragile, she was not a candidate for weekly visits to the dialysis center. Instead, she had tubing surgically implanted into her abdomen for dialysis at home, four times a day.

Her rapidly failing lungs required her to begin using oxygen. Soon, she was in a wheelchair. Next, I had a hospital bed placed in our bedroom because she couldn't breathe lying down. Shortly after that, I had to call for an ambulance to rush her to the local hospital after a "spell." She had lost consciousness at home and I feared the worst. By the time I arrived at the hospital, Sue was being rushed to emergency surgery. Her pericardium, the sac around her heart, had filled with fluid. Neither her kidneys nor the dialysis worked. After the surgery, I was told that they drained fifteen hundred cc's of fluid from a space that normally held fifty cc's. During the next week, Sue didn't bounce back as she normally did. She slowly recovered from the operation and I took her home.

Six weeks before Sue's final hospitalization, I helped her visit another local hospital. She wasn't there as a patient this time. She was in her wheelchair with an oxygen tank and other equipment she required in tow. She wasn't there for medical treatment. She was there to visit her new granddaughter, Bailey May Curtis. I believe that brief visit did more for Sue that any medical care she could have received. I took many pictures of the two of them together. I knew what Sue was thinking. She was probably saying to herself, "I wish I could be around to take care of this little bundle and watch her grow."

The final five weeks of Sue's life are still a blur to me. During this period of time, Sue's body literally filled up with fluid. I would sit at night with her on the couch, and I had to put at least four inches of toweling under her feet to catch the water flowing from the pores in her legs. Soon, she was unable to bend her legs because of the fluid. Eventually, the fluid reached as high as her waist. She was drowning on the inside.

The week before Sue died; I announced to the public that I would not be running for another term as mayor of our town. I did so, at that time, because nominating petitions were due, and I had to let people who were supporting me know what I was doing. I said that getting Sue back on her feet was my first priority, period.

Two local newspapers picked up on the story, and one asked if they could come and get a picture of Sue and me together and interview us. We were both public figures in our community. I asked Sue if she approved and she said, "Sure, but I'll have to get my hair done!" That was typical of Sue.

The reporter and photographer arrived, took Sue's picture and interviewed us. For a while during the interview, Sue was her old self. That weekend, both papers ran a front-page story with a head and shoulders picture of Sue with a big smile. Other than for a few close friends, no one really knew how sick she was. After the article appeared, cards and calls of well-wishers started to come in, many of them from people Sue had helped over the years. She enjoyed hearing from them.

Sue's final trip to the hospital soon followed. She had emergency surgery to remove another two thousand cc's of fluid from around her heart. She never recovered from that operation. When her friends arrived at the hospital from Grand Rapids, the same couple who had been with us at the Traverse City restaurant that Labor Day weekend, Sue looked at them and said, "Well, this is it." She didn't have much to say after that. For a few days she drifted in and out of consciousness surrounded by close friends and family.

When Sue's struggle appeared to be lost, I asked her doctor to meet with my daughters and me. I read him the following statement that Sue had placed in her directive for final medical care. She had written: "Please, when you see that the end of my life is near, don't try any heroic efforts to prolong it."

In many ways, Sue was a very complex person, but on that point she wanted to be absolutely clear. I knew, and my daughters agreed, that Sue had reached that final point where there was nothing to be done. Her doctor said that he understood and doubted that Sue would regain consciousness. Subsequently, I signed the necessary legal papers, life support apparatus was removed, and the next day, August 13, 1999, Sue died.

Traverse City Record-Eagle
Susan (Hartwick) Bailey
Died August 13, 1999

Susan (Hartwick) Bailey, of Flushing and Interlochen, died Friday at McLaren Regional Medical Center in Flint. Born in Grand Rapids, she was the daughter of Harold and Gladys (Pease) Hartwick. In 1957, in Grand Rapids, she married Archie Bailey. Susan graduated from Michigan State University and completed graduate work at Oakland University.

She was a thirty-five-year summer resident of Interlochen, spending summers at Pennlock Colony on Green Lake raising children and grandchildren.

She was also a dedicated public servant who held a variety of appointed and elected offices. She served on the Oakland County Board of Supervisors, the Flushing City Council and the Flushing Planning Board.

She was a five-term Genesee County commissioner and officer of the Michigan Association of Counties. Susan also served as Genesee County's Chief Deputy County Clerk.

As a member of the Genesee County Parks and Recreation Commission, she is credited with having helped to create the concept of holding an annual Christmas festival at Crossroads Village, now known as Christmas at Crossroads, a popular annual event in mid-Michigan. Michigan Governor, James Blanchard, appointed Susan to the Michigan Sesquicentennial Commission, the Community Corrections Board and the Local Government Claims and Review Board.

She retired from public life in 1992, but she continued to be active in organizations committed to the welfare of children. For thirteen years, she served on and chaired the Genesee County Substance Abuse Commission and the Newpaths Board of Directors.

Most recently, she was appointed by the Michigan State Supreme Court to the State Foster Care Review Board.

She is survived by her husband, Archie; daughters, Katherine (Kevin) Bailey-Curtis and Sarah Marie Coyner; and beloved grandchildren, Brandon, Bradley, Erica, and newly arrived Bailey May Curtis.

Cremation has taken place. A memorial service was held at 4 P.M. Monday, at the Flushing Presbyterian Church. Memorial contributions in her memory may be directed to the Humane Society of Genesee County, PO Box 190138, Burton, MI 48519. Arrangements were handled by Rossell Funeral Home in Flushing.

Personnel of the local funeral home told me later that Sue's funeral was the largest in Flushing's history. She was a lifelong Episcopalian, but the local Episcopal Church wasn't large enough to hold the large turnout, so the service was held in our town's larger Presbyterian Church. Sue would have appreciated that kind of ecumenical cooperation.

The weeks before and after Sue's death are still almost a total blur to me. As I look back now at some of the things written and said about Sue at the time of her death, I get a much clearer picture of the role she played in many lives, in many ways.

Sue served for many years on Genesee County's Substance Abuse Commission. She had to resign from the Commission because of her illness. The evening she retired, the Substance Abuse Commission honored her. They said, "Sue Bailey, this one's for you. This evening the Board and staff have chosen to honor you in a very special way.

"Over many years you have always been there for all of us and especially for those served by the Substance Abuse Commission. Your relationship started many years ago when you were a member of the Youth Assistance Board in Flushing. You continued your involvement as a member of the County Board of Commissioners. Even as chairperson of the County Board of Commissioners, you took extra time to become the commissioners' representative.

"For thirteen years you have served us well in times of plenty and in times of dissension. At no time have you served us better than in the past year. Sue, you have been the advocate, administrator, president, facilitator, the glue, the inspiration, and the encourager.

"You never back away from a fight, but you never forget to acknowledge the positive, and you are truly a friend indeed to all of us and we are indebted to you. You are a living example of how one person can make a difference, a personal philosophy that we know you believe in.

"Your personal and professional life is an exemplification of the phrase with those ten two-letter words: If it is to be, it is up to me."

A reporter expressed it another way in an interview a few days before Sue's death. She said to me, "Mayor Bailey, you have your supporters and critics, but I have never heard anyone say anything negative about Sue Bailey."

At her funeral, the Episcopal minister quoted from a poem that he said summed up what Susan Bailey meant to the lives of those people she touched. He said, "Some people come into our lives and go quickly, but others leave footprints on our hearts and we will never be the same. Many of you will share footprints she left on your heart."

A state representative who knew Sue well said, "She was a mentor for women just getting into politics and a role model for us all."

An Associated Press story reporting Sue's death included the following comment from a former county commissioner, who had served with Sue: "She was one of the major women members of the county Board of

Commissioners. She provided a leadership role model for a number of women like myself."

The "stand-in" who took on Sue's case during her first hospitalization was impressed with Sue's ability to deal with his staff. The title of "stand-in" was soon changed to "the good shepherd." He was the director of the Family Practice Residency Program and supervised the medical education of all his students. She labeled him "the good shepherd" because he rarely came into her room or saw her in the office alone. He was always surrounded by medical students who seemed to hover around him and follow him up and down the hospital's halls like so many sheep. He guided them with great care.

After Sue's death, he wrote the following to me: "I hope you realize that I appreciated Susan not only as a person and a patient but as a very fine teacher of medicine in her very own right. She was always kind and very patient with the many learners she saw, and I think that she probably understood her important role in educating them about her illness and enhancing their abilities to diagnose and treat other people who may suffer the same or similar afflictions. Many of the medical residents who saw her, expressed their gratitude, if not to her, then to me, for her kindness, patience, and wisdom in sharing her experiences so freely with them."

The accolades continued to come in for Sue after her death. In July, the Flushing Concerts in the Park Series was dedicated to her memory. The family established the *Susan H. Bailey Spartan Scholarship* pledging twenty-five one-thousand-dollar scholarships over twenty-five years. A plaque was placed in the local library in her honor.

Originally, I was asked by an online scleroderma awareness organization to write "Scleroderma: Sue's Story" so that others with scleroderma could get as inclusive a picture of scleroderma as possible. The condition of every scleroderma patient is different. Somewhere, to someone, Sue's story may offer some insight into his or her own case.

Since I began writing, however, I have decided that "Scleroderma: Sue's Story" could provide interesting reading for our grandchildren, especially Bailey May, who never got to know her grandmother. For that reason, I have added some biographical information about their wonderful grandmother that may be useful to them, someday, as they tell Sue's story to their children.

◆ ❖ ◆

Christine L. Beck
Surviving Daughter of Veta Breit
Illinois, USA

I am very proud of the fight my mother put up. She lived fourteen years with CREST scleroderma. She died on June 9, 1999. She died a terrible death.

She handled the disease very well for the pain she was in, but eventually it took her away from me. She got to where she couldn't even enjoy bingo, which she dearly loved. We live in cold weather, which affected her hands and feet.

She was the most wonderful mother and friend I could have ever had. And she was one of the bravest women I ever saw. When she was diagnosed with CREST, she was very scared. For the longest time she tried to get help so that she could understand what was wrong with her. It took a long time. She finally had a blood test done that revealed it.

She saw a doctor in Rockford who was wonderful. My mother had the hardening of the skin, and ulcers on her hands, feet and, ears. She had difficulty swallowing and hoarseness. In the end, her insides hardened as well as her outside, right before our very eyes! It was the most awful death I had ever seen.

She could not breathe at the end. She was on quite a lot of medication and nothing helped. She went and pushed on for years until it finally won. The cold got to be too much for her. Even her smoking got to be too much.

She had a very strong will about her and she pushed her self to the limit. I only hope I am as strong a person as she was. She was my very best friend. She was there for me when I buried my twenty-two-year-old son, and I was there for her until the end. The world and I lost a great woman and friend. I am very proud of the fight she put up.

I now wonder if I have it in my hands and feet as they turn very bluish black, and I get very hoarse now and then and seem to be very tired a lot.

I have a lot of heartburn. I had a blood test done a few years ago and they say, "no." But another doctor says I have Raynaud's phenomenon. I can't stand the cold or putting my hands in the freezer. My hands hurt and get cramped sometimes when they get cold. Can someone help me?

◆ ❖ ◆

Jamie Valentine
Surviving Spouse
New Jersey, USA

My husband Jerry was diagnosed with scleroderma at age thirty-five in January 2000. He was told that he had Raynaud's phenomenon in October 1999 and was sent to a specialist who diagnosed the scleroderma. Prior to the Raynaud's diagnosis, he was fairly healthy, but he began to lose weight and complained of stiffness in his knees. Not in a million years did we think his scleroderma would progress so quickly.

In April 2000, we went to the hospital because he had shortness of breath. We were told that he had heart failure and pneumonia, and he began a series of medications to prevent the heart from failing.

In July 2000, he also began treatment for scleroderma again. His scleroderma doctor in Philadelphia told us that he had good news and bad news. The good news was that we came to him and could possibly "catch up" to the disease. The bad news was that it was progressing rapidly. My husband used to take over seven different medications a day. This was terrible on the psyche of a man who was very active and considerably healthy prior to all of this.

To make a long story short, he had terrible pain in his hands from August until he passed away on October 23, 2000. He went to the hospital with shortness of breath and he was told that he had pneumonia again and that his heart had deteriorated even more. His cause of death was listed as cardiac arrest, pneumonia, and scleroderma.

This is a terrible disease for anyone—even your worst enemy. The pain in his hands was so bad that he used to say it would knock him out. He was still employed as a teacher and managed to drive to work, although my children and I couldn't understand how he did it.

I just want to say that my husband was courageous in many ways, even though he lost the battle. He was confident that a cure would be found in his lifetime that would help others. The disease is so peculiar that I still question whether or not more immediate attention should be given to research for a cure. I am anxious because no one knows if it is hereditary or not, and my children still have to grow up. I am thankful for the ISN's website for allowing others to share their stories. I tried on many occasions to find more awareness through other websites such as this one. I hope more men will post their stories because scleroderma is rare in men.

◆ ❖ ◆

Keenan Jennings
Surviving Son of Fibrosing Alveolitis Patient
Peru

Dad passed away now almost four years ago. It still hurts knowing that I will never be able to ask his advice or listen to his corny jokes again. He was just fifty-eight years old.

Although Dad was a heavy smoker for much of his life, I am told that the fibrosing alveolitis that killed him could not be directly related to this. In fact, nothing could be directly related and, indeed, it took some time to diagnose the problem.

The end came relatively rapidly. From the time of initial diagnosis, there were eighteen short months. The disease got worse, rendering it a chore for dad to even walk to the mailbox. The steroids helped very little and, in the end, ever-increasing doses of morphine meant he lost some of his lucidity. It is a cruel disease, with no cure. The scarring gets worse, and the shortness of breath more desperate. Finally dad succumbed and was released from the ever-harder battle to simply breathe.

It is tough to write about, but cathartic as well. I miss him a lot and wish that I could have just a little more time to tell him how much I love him.

Lung diseases are dreadful, but I hope that the experts continue their research so that our loved ones can live easier and longer.

Krista Lurtz
Father's Passing
Romania

We all know how hard it is to cope with the emotional side of an incurable disease. After months of surfing the Internet, stubborn to find a break in the disease, I didn't give up when I realized that there was nothing to do to cure myself.

After many nights of tears, I decided to start the translation of the www.sclero.org web pages. I've realized that this way I can help myself and I can also help others, both patients and caregivers. The only help that we can give is emotional help. That is all. I was a caregiver and now I am a patient. Today, I will write my caregiver story for you, because that was what made me start the Romanian translation of this website.

Unfortunately, my father was sick for seven years. He had different problems (work-related illness) with his lungs, his heart, and diabetes. All those years beside him, seeing him suffer, being frustrated about the fact that I could not do anything to help him, I went through all the emotions that come with that: the grief, the sorrow, and all the nights witnessing his tears and prayers to take his life away, because he was suffering so much. It was not a life for him anymore. There was only the oxygen installation to help him.

If scleroderma needs a trigger, the trigger for me was the night when my father died. I am sure about that. Emotionally, it was too much for me. I loved him more than anything in the world. We were very close, and we had so much in common. He was my first dance and music teacher; my best friend; the one who taught me to love the mountains, the animals, the forest, cooking; laughing; and having a lot of fun.

I can say, without making any mistakes, that I am a copy of my father, especially when it comes to talking about a sense of humor (and being stubborn.) He was a very strong person. He taught me to go through life fighting and not to give up! He never did. With love, and deep respect for my father, I will not give up, no matter how my life is: bad or good.

Yes, I must say, he gave me the fighting spirit and he taught me that with a good laugh you can go on, even if that laughter comes along with tears.

On that night he died, I was there with my mom. It was a very cold February night. It was my mom who called to tell me, "Your father wants to see you and his grandson Alex."

I didn't wait. I took my son and I went to my parents' place, our old and beloved house. When I saw the look in his eyes, I knew that he would die that night. Something inside me told me that on that night, I would witness life and death. I had so many tears inside me, but I could not cry in front of him. I knew he would not like that, and my tears would hurt him so much. He was so strong, and I felt that if I cried that night, I would be letting him down! So I let my tears cry inside of me.

Late in the night, sitting beside him, he started having moments when he didn't realize where he was. At those moments, he started calling with a voice that I always will hear in my mind: "Krista, my dear, please take me home!"

He was breaking my heart. I wanted to scream against life, against death, against all the gods in the sky, no matter what their names were. But I could not. I had to be strong. I held his hand and wiped his face with a wet towel. That was all I could do.

Behind those tears, I put the screams. I kept everything inside me. The only thought on my mind in those moments, holding his hand, was my prayer, "God, please release him! If you want someone to suffer, and if someone must suffer for an unknown reason (something that only you know, God), please give me the suffering, but release him! Give me all his pain, but let him go. Take him home, and take care of him. He has had enough!"

I never prayed harder and with all my soul than in those moments, for nothing. That was my strongest prayer that I ever said, and it was my scream against something that I feel was very unfair. Everything was inside me. It was a lot of pressure, but I could not let it out.

In those moments when he was coherent, he was telling me jokes. That was my father, the one who used to make jokes about the terrible moments in his life. Sitting on that line, between life and death, I saw him passing away, with his forehead up, with his fighting spirit up. I learned my last lesson from him. My first teacher in my life, who taught me to walk, was now teaching me how to die. Between those two lessons, he taught me how to live, how to go on, how to fight, and never to give up!

Early in the morning, he said that he would go home in the daylight. He only wanted to go home, and get some rest, because he was feeling very tired. At 8:15, outside, the snow was shining, touched by the first sunlight shine, when he quietly passed away.

It was like I was frozen inside. Time had stopped, somehow, in me. I had no other reaction. In my mind was: "He is fine now. He finally found his peace, and he is resting now. I must be strong. I must stay beside him, until he is grieved. I have a lot of time to cry, later on. Not now."

So I didn't cry, and I didn't scream. But I felt all the pressure inside of me, localized in one point on my back. It was becoming a physical pain for me. From that moment, that pain never stopped. It is always there, and my condition is getting worse, every day.

I have moments when I have many questions: "Did that happen? Did God listen to my prayers, and did He do what I was asking Him to? Did I help my father with that? Am I the one who inherits his suffering?" After all, I had asked for it.

My answer for this is: "Whatever happened, I know I did the right thing." If someone will tell me one day, "Yes, you are suffering because you agreed to take over all his pains, and you were praying for that!" I would still not feel sorry for what I've done. I would do it again today, if I could turn back the hands of time.

For many years, I was feeling the grief that I could not help him. Many times I wanted to give years of my life to help him, if that was the price. My love for him will never die. I know that he is always beside me, with his spirit, and thinking of him, I find my strength to go on. I know that I am doing the right thing. If I've taken over his pain, I've also taken over his strength. I will do it the way he did it. I will fight, and I will smile.

I'm not saying that life is always fair with me, or that I don't have moments when I feel completely lost or scared. I'm not saying that I don't have moments when I'm losing the sense of life. All that I am saying is that the only way to go on is to keep on fighting in the first place, with your own self.

Now perhaps you can better understand why I started to translate this website. Why did I start such a difficult job, when it was so hard for me? When you deal with pain, it is hard to do anything else.

I am a very logical person, and I was thinking this way: It was not my choice to live a life like this. I did not want to be this way. I felt a lot of pain living beside my father those years. I'm going through a lot of pain now because of my new condition. I must live on with my past and my present. I do not look that much for the future. I've learned to live for today.

I do not consider myself lucky that I've had the caregiver experience, but I can put both of my experiences together and I can help people see both sides of this kind of story. Or, at least I can try to do that.

I am not giving advice; I just want you to know the way I feel. And I've learned that when you find a person who feels the same as you, they will help you understand yourself better.

Whether you are a patient or a caregiver, your life has been changed; it is no longer normal. You become more concerned about everyone around you. Emotionally, you become too sensitive. Your way of thinking about life has changed, and nobody can feel things the same as you.

Another lesson that I've learned from my father is: "Whatever you do, think about the people around you. Try not to bother them, and go on with what you want to do. Make sure that you don't hurt anyone, and believe in what you are doing. Believe in yourself."

Since I've had the certitude that I have three incurable diseases, my life has changed. I am more concerned about the other people that are suffering. I'm going to do the best that I can to help in every way I can. I feel very limited sometimes, because I want to help more and more.

My Romanian translation has many pages because I added a lot of articles that I hope will help others dealing emotionally with the situation. We can't say a lot about medical things, but we can help emotionally.

What if I am thinking now that life is unfair with me? Unfair is when someone is suffering like this. But, what is fair? It is not fair for the sun to be covered with clouds! It is not fair that children are living in this world in terrible conditions. It is not fair that there is war around the world. There are so many things that are unfair.

Today, writing this for you (this is my first time writing in English), I realized that when I was a caregiver, I missed the best thing to do for myself, to help myself to understand my father better: I should have read about the emotional changes in a person who is living every day of their life in pain.

My thought for caregivers now is: If you learn about a disease, you can better understand what it is happening with us. On the other hand, we don't talk every day about the pain. If I start complaining about every pain in my body, who will stay beside me? And probably I would not have time for any other conversation. Why? Because, it hurts! For five minutes the pain is in my leg, the next five minutes it hurts in my shoulder, and after another five minutes, the pain is somewhere in my kidneys! Try to imagine a person who is complaining all day long, about so many kinds of pain—skin burning or muscles tingling. (Personally, I don't think that I could complain like that!)

Learning about it, you would eliminate from the beginning the questions: "Do you have pain now? Are you okay?"

If I am laughing, it does not mean I am without pain. It just means I am laughing. If I am sitting at the table at dinner and I start crying when, for others, there is nothing to cry over, it means that my throat refuses to let the food go down, or that it is very painful to swallow.

How can I not cry? What is in my mind at that point? "I am thirty-one years old! If I cannot control this, what else do I expect to do?" It is grief! Why do I cry when I am walking upstairs in the house? Because I am thinking, "I used to climb mountains. Now, to walk up the stairs one level in my house, it takes all the energy out of me!"

And there are so many other things that I am thinking about. I used to be a great dancer; I can't do that anymore. I used to love to walk into the forest; I can't do that anymore. I use to play with children a lot of the time; I do not have that energy anymore.

Yes, I am thirty-one years old. I have had to give up a lot of things, but I will never give up fighting with my new condition. This summer, when I go home to Romania, I hope to take a walk in the forest, and in the mountains, and to have a lovely night dancing. I will do it, but not like in the old times.

LaVonne Carson
Surviving Mother of a Daughter with MCTD
British Columbia, Canada

I'm the mother of an only daughter who had mixed connective tissue disease (MCTD). She died in March 2000 at thirty-five years of age.

She was diagnosed with MCTD in 1996. She went into an emergency room in California on March 16 with a little fluid around her heart. They sent her home with a shot of morphine and prednisone, and told her to come back if she got worse.

She slept all day and could not feel any pain to know she was getting worse. Her husband decided to take her back to the hospital around four o'clock that afternoon. They got two miles from their house and she said, "Kev, something is seriously wrong," and fell over in the Jeep. She had no pulse.

By the time the ambulance arrived to take her to the hospital, her heart had stopped. They got it going and drained off all the fluid from around her heart. Both the medics and her husband, Kevin, used cardiopulmonary resuscitation (CPR) but unfortunately, the fluid had prevented it from working. So she was, basically, brain dead by the side of the road, and they had only six miles more to get to the hospital.

The reason I'm writing this is to say that if any of you out there have MCTD, lupus, scleroderma, etc., please don't take your symptoms lightly. I have no faith in doctors anymore. I can't understand why they didn't keep my daughter in the hospital that morning when she went into the emergency room at two o'clock in the morning. They could have simply monitored her for twenty-four hours, and they would have seen she was in trouble with the extra fluid accumulating around her heart. Then, they could have drained it off like they did later, and she would still be with us today.

She had a wonderful career going at age thirty-five and was teaching the dental hygiene program at UCSF as well as doing research there also. I miss her so much, and I also miss the fact that she didn't get to give me grandchildren. That's what she wanted most, to have a baby, which they were planning.

I would like to hear from anyone else out there that has been diagnosed with MCTD. I would like to know more about it and your symptoms. Thank you, and God bless each and every one of you.

◆ ❖ ◆

Marie Carey
Surviving Spouse of Scleroderma Patient
Arizona, USA

My name is Marie, and my husband died one and a half years ago from progressive systemic scleroderma.

When Dean and I married, he was a healthy and fit man of thirty-three, working in the sand and gravel industry. After our first year of marriage, he became increasingly more tired and achy as the days passed by. It took one year of multiple misdiagnoses before it was determined that he had scleroderma.

He kept on working as he progressively got worse. Scleroderma affected every part of his body. Dean was a strong-willed "redneck" man and was never able to accept the severity of his disease. We went through a half dozen doctors until we found the last set, and they took good care of him until the end.

For me, the hardest part was watching him suffer in pain and not being able to help him. We tried numerous things to help him, from holistic medicine to an electrical stimulator placed in his spine to generate blood flow. Poor Dean was stuck and tested so many times then.

Towards the end, he was improving. We placed him on a twenty-four-hour intravenous (IV) bag to feed him and help him gain weight. He started moving around again and we took his kids to San Diego for a weekend at Sea World and the beach.

Upon our return two days later, he contracted an infection. The doctors told me he had a staph infection, spinal meningitis, pneumonia, and his heart was going ballistic. Four days later he died quietly and peacefully while holding my hand. He was finally free from suffering.

Dean left me as well as his two children behind, but we have survived. I can only say to other loved ones that, indeed, it was the hardest thing I have ever gone through. Just hang in there and let God take you through it. Of the six years I was married to him, he was healthy only one year. But I am so glad and proud to have been his wife.

◆ ❖ ◆

Sonya D. Bethea
Surviving Daughter-in-Law
South Carolina, USA

This is in loving memory of CB. My mother-in-law was diagnosed about two years ago with diffuse scleroderma with CREST. It all started with a small patch of dark, hardened skin on her upper back. Concerned over the patch, she decided to see her physician, who referred her to a dermatologist, who referred her to a specialist, and so on and so forth.

After several months of referrals, she received her diagnosis. Initially, my mother-in-law was told that she would be fine as long as the disease didn't spread to her internal organs. She was told to avoid stress as stress accelerates the disease.

Last year, CB was forced to leave her job to go on disability. Since that time, I've watched her change from being a beautiful woman, full of life, into what seems like a one-hundred-year-old person with the inability to do anything for herself. This is especially difficult for her because she is the type of person who has always been very meticulous about her appearance. Her hair, nails, and clothes were always perfect. She enjoyed shopping as well as vacationing several times a year in Las Vegas.

I cannot believe that she is the same person. I have watched her health decline very rapidly in the last year. CB cannot feed herself, comb her hair, go to the bathroom, or even turn herself over in bed. She has lost so much weight that her skin is literally hanging like a pair of stockings that are four or five sizes too large.

Although CB and I haven't always been as close as I would have liked, it breaks my heart to see her this way. Her quality of life is zero. The really sad part is that many of our family members, ministers, and friends are telling her that she is going to get better, that a miracle is going to happen and she will be her old self again.

I think that we all need to give her permission to die. I believe CB is hanging on for everyone else. I think we should let her know that it is okay to die. I would rather relish the memory of her before this debilitating disease ravishes her body.

In October of 2000, doctors told CB that she had a few days, weeks, or a month to live. She is still with us. Two weeks ago, the hospice stated that if she lived until the end of this month, it would be a miracle.

I think scleroderma is, in many ways, worse than cancer. This disease totally strips a person of their independence and dignity. I never thought that

I would, literally, have to hand CB a drink of water or aid with toileting.

Update

My mother-in-law's health has further deteriorated. She has been taken off all medication with the exception of pain meds. She no longer eats or communicates. Every now and then, when she hears a familiar voice, she opens her eyes. Although her eyes are open, I don't think she sees anyone. As I lie on the bed beside her and gently rub her hand, I find myself not recognizing her. This is not my mother-in-law.

I struggle to remember her beauty before scleroderma and to remember her last words before she stopped communicating. The image of the beautiful woman, once engraved in my memory, is slowly being replaced with the image of this very sick person whose life hangs by a mere thread. This deeply disturbs me because it is not the image I want to remain once she is gone.

The nurse says that death is near. I look at her and wonder how much sicker a person can possibly get before death occurs. I can't describe the feeling I get seeing her so helpless and ill. I long to hear her speak—just once more. I want to tell her that I love her and will see her again one day.

One of CB's sisters came home from New York yesterday and told CB not to worry about the family. That was her way of saying it was okay to leave us. She had the courage to say what the rest of the family had not been able to say. We all love her and, if given a choice, would want her to be her old self again, but we all realize that's not going to happen. None of us wants to continue seeing her this way.

Update

On May 7, 2001, scleroderma took CB from us. My husband, a sister, and both of CB's parents were by her side. I am thankful that CB no longer suffers and that she is with God, but words cannot describe how much I miss her. My heart is broken.

My father-in-law said that he told CB to do what she had to and that he would be okay. He said approximately twenty minutes later, she died. I guess she needed to know that the family would be okay before she could leave us.

My husband said CB died peacefully. I saw her shortly after she died. As she died at home, she was a vision of loveliness! All of the blemishes left her face, and her skin was soft and radiant. She didn't look as if she was ever ill, so I like to think that CB now has eternal health and peace.

◆ ❖ ◆

Star
Surviving Spouse
Virginia, USA

My name is Star and I want to share my story about my husband. I am forty-three and I lost my husband on October 7, 2001. He had scleroderma for two years.

We were married for twenty-four years and have three sons ages twentyone, twenty-two, and twenty-four. He was very strong man, a loving husband, and father.

Frankie was my life, whom I love and will never forget, but he gave me strength to continue, and if I can help someone like you and give you strength to go on with life, then I know he's smiling on me.

William Jordan
Surviving Boyfriend
Alabama, USA

Wendy Carter passed away in July of 1998 after a long, courageous battle against systemic scleroderma, lupus, and pulmonary hypertension—all complicated by diabetes.

I met Wendy in July of 1997 when she was only in her fourth month of coming to terms with her illness. In March of that year, her doctors told her that she could hope for only three to five years of life remaining. But the clock was ticking much faster than anyone realized at the time.

On our initial date, I experienced the first of many burdens that come with being close to a scleroderma patient. Wendy was heart-set on dancing that evening, even though she was connected to an oxygen machine by a fifty-foot cord. We took the machine with us and managed to "cut the rug" in spite of the difficulties. That was when I realized that there was more life left in Wendy than in a lot of people who take their good health for granted. She had won me over, and the joys that she brought me easily began to overtake the inconveniences.

Wendy found solace in her large, caring family that extended from Mobile, Alabama, and the surrounding communities to the Macon, Georgia, area where she grew up. Most of all, she cherished moments spent with her children in Georgia, either on the phone, or during the special times they were able to be together. Though she was unable to care for them on a daily basis, her love for them was unconquerable.

During the fall of last year, Wendy's condition worsened, and the hospital became an increasingly familiar environment for her. By the time of a long-awaited New Year's trip to the Smoky Mountains, Raynaud's phenomenon, a complication of Wendy's scleroderma, had begun its horrible assault on her hands, resulting in the amputation of two fingers the following spring. Wendy was losing weight and her health, but not her faith or her determination to make the best of her situation.

My love for Wendy grew steadily, and her family and I tried to help her achieve some satisfaction and happiness in the days she had left. But her illnesses would not wait, and she passed away peacefully at home amidst her family in the twilight of a warm, July day. Her legacy lives on in her children and the memories and love she left behind. We will always love Wendy.

◆ ❖ ◆

PART 2

Juvenile and Localized Scleroderma

CHAPTER 5

Juvenile Scleroderma

Can you please help me find a cure
by starting Juvenile Scleroderma research?.

— B. J. Gaither

Juvenile Scleroderma
Medical Overview of Juvenile Scleroderma (JSD)
By Thomas J. A. Lehman M.D., F.A.A.P., F.A.C.R.

Dr. Lehman is Chief of the Division of Pediatric Rheumatology for The Hospital for Special Surgery, and Professor of Clinical Pediatrics at Cornell University Medical Center in New York.

Whenever any form of scleroderma begins during childhood, it is also called juvenile scleroderma. From the physician's point of view, taking care of children with scleroderma is a source of both great satisfaction and great distress. It is very satisfying to care for children with linear or focal scleroderma. The majority of children do extremely well. Those who have significant involvement are often dramatically improved by methotrexate therapy. Watching a child's skin become softer and the areas of contractures improve is an extremely satisfying experience. Once the area has improved, it is very unlikely that the problem will recur.

It is also extremely pleasing to see children with progressive systemic sclerosis (PSS) improve with therapy; however, this is a chronic disease and much more challenging from the physician's viewpoint. So far there is no cure for PSS; however, we can make children dramatically better. This should make it easy for physicians. Current medications make it easy for physicians to slow the progression of scleroderma. If a child's disease is mild to moderate, we appear to be able to partially reverse it and dramatically slow its progress. But we cannot undo extensive damage, and it is not certain that we can stop the disease completely.

As a physician, I feel so much frustration when I see a child with PSS who has had the disease for many years, yet has not been aggressively treated. If the disease is far advanced, slowing it down is not going to be enough. Over the years, I have shared the remaining time and ultimate grief with many families of children with PSS. This is never an easy thing for a physician. In some ways it was easier in the past. Twenty-five years ago, there was little hope for a child with PSS. With recent progress, we do so much better. That makes it much harder for me to see a child who has severe advanced disease that is beyond what I can hope to fix.

Even more challenging for physicians are the children who receive therapy, improve, and then do not want to continue the treatment. Weekly or biweekly shots of methotrexate are no fun. Many children feel ill the day after the injection. When the child has obvious disease and everyone sees the improvement, they are willing to put up with the inconvenience. When they get better, they want to stop. Unfortunately, PSS often starts to come back when they stop. As a physician, it is my job to convince people that they need to keep getting shots they do not want. Often, families decide to stop and say they will restart therapy if they see the disease coming back. Unfortunately, it often does. However, when I immediately want the child to restart the medication, there is often resistance.

How should a physician approach family members or children with PSS who do not want to continue or restart therapy? Is it fair to show pictures of children with terrible disease and say this is what used to happen to everyone, and it will happen to you? Probably not! Is it fair to let the families avoid therapy knowing that the child probably will do badly in the end? Probably not! So what do you do? There is only one thing you can really do. You inform the families about your experience, and you encourage them to make the right choice. Some do, some do not. You have to be there for both.

In twenty-five years of practicing pediatric rheumatology, I have seen linear and focal scleroderma become very treatable and dramatically reversible diseases. I have seen many smiles and many dramatic improvements. I have seen PSS change from a steadily worsening condition to one that I can at least partially reverse. The healing skin and increased energy bring great pleasure to the families and to me.

I hope that with greater awareness and understanding, more children will receive early aggressive care. If we can accomplish that goal, we will have made great progress. After that, we need to learn how to make families realize that care must continue after the children look well. If we can do that, perhaps we can claim to have truly changed the outcome.

B. J. Gaither
California, USA

I am eleven years old and I have juvenile scleroderma (JSD). Having JSD has limited me to what I can do and not do as far as being like other kids. I cannot run around the school like the other kids. Sometimes I need help opening up my milk. I cannot write as fast or as long when I am trying to do my class work or homework. It hurts to carry my backpack. Sometimes when my mom picks me up from school, I can barely walk to the car. It really is awful having something wrong with you and trying to be like all the other kids at school or in your neighborhood.

Having JSD makes me feel angry. I am tired of getting blood tests every month for the past seven years. I am tired of the kids making fun of me. Sometimes they call me "surgery boy" or they say, "Oh, he's the boy with arthritis! We can twist his arm and break it." I have too many doctors' appointments and take too much medicine that does not make me feel very good.

Sometimes my mom will say, "If we could turn back time..." Well, I would like to go forward to the last day of my life so I could die and start a new life without JSD. I feel this way because JSD makes me mad and sad. It is stupid to have JSD because it causes me to hurt inside and outside.

If I could, I would get rid of JSD by making a video game device inside your body that you could use to zap the bad germs to make it go away!

I want researchers and the government to find a cure by looking at the air, plants, forest, and snow; to see what is good and bad; to identify different diseases; and to know how to take care of it so that in a couple of weeks, it would be gone. If we cannot find a cure, I just want to die. Can you please help me find a cure by starting JSD research?

◆ ❖ ◆

Debbie Lyndon
Daughter Bregan, Morphea
New Zealand

I am a mother of six children. My fourth child, Bregan, who is seven years old, has just been diagnosed with morphea. This started three years ago with a patch on the left side of her abdomen, and it seems to be spreading around the left side to her back. She is still going for blood tests to make sure it is not affecting any other body organs.

This is all new to me, and I am finding it hard to understand. I have a lot of questions, but find it hard to get the answers. I suppose you could say I am hoping for good answers to say that this is just going to go away.

We live in New Zealand and have been told this is very rare. Bregan has seen several specialists, and they were a bit skeptical at first, but I think it is because they do not know enough about it.

Could someone please tell me more about it and help me understand this disease a bit more?

Dot
Son Cole, Morphea/Linear
Missouri, USA

In September of 2000, we noticed a discoloration of skin on our son's elbow and forearm. I thought it was from sunburn and was just peeling. In October, I noticed that the discoloration was growing larger, and it was shiny and hairless.

Around Halloween, we took Cole to our regular family doctor who immediately thought it was scleroderma and sent us to a dermatologist. She took one look and said she thought, for sure, it was morphea. We went in for a skin biopsy and are still awaiting results.

The dermatologist said there is no cure or treatment, although she would like to see Cole in physical therapy so he will not lose movement in his arm.

I have read many of the stories posted on the www.sclero.org website and have felt encouraged by them. Cole really has not experienced any pain or limitations yet. I hope it does not appear anywhere else on him. Any advice would be helpful. This is all new for us.

Update – February 2001

Cole was diagnosed with morphea/linear. We have been seeing a pediatric dermatologist. She has Cole on steroid cream. It has shown a little improvement already. The skin does not seem to be as tight. So we are just taking this a day at a time.

Jane
Daughter Jenny, Morphea
Texas, USA

In 1990, my healthy and bright six-year-old daughter, Jenny, complained that her right foot was itching and hurting. Soon after, dark spots mixed with white patches appeared on her foot. Her back, just below her armpit, and the front of her right thigh began to show the same patchiness. Her foot began to contract and became difficult for her to straighten.

The doctor said it appeared to be morphea, and possibly, scleroderma. I immediately searched for any information I could find, but to no avail. There was very little information back then, even in the library. The doctor explained that it was a disease in white women usually between the ages of thirty-five and fifty. He described systemic scleroderma with the tightening of the skin which usually began with the hands and then moved on to other parts of the body with the organs coming last. The ultimate prognosis: death.

We were horrified but told not to worry. Not all cases are extreme and because Jenny was so young, she would probably have a better chance. The only correlation we found was a tick bite Jenny had received three weeks before the first appearance of morphea. She was on an Indian Princess camp-out with her father, and although he pulled the tick out of her back (right side), the tick's head remained. We eventually prayed over Jenny with our minister asking for healing and that the morphea would stop. And it did.

My daughter is now fifteen, still bright, but has been left with some permanent, brown scarring on her leg, foot, and back. Our doctor recently gave her some bleaching cream to try to restore some of the color, because it is visible when Jenny wears a bathing suit. She has forgotten a lot about the morphea, but I have not.

About the same time Jenny was diagnosed with morphea, she began to lose some of her hearing. She now has fifty percent loss in one ear and a thirty-five percent loss in the other. I cannot help but wonder if there is some correlation. Is hearing loss associated with morphea? Her hearing specialist has asked this question because we cannot find any other cause. She had perfect hearing prior to age six and no traumas. I am particularly concerned with the reccurrence of morphea, or the possibility of systemic scleroderma. I was happy to learn that morphea usually does not recur, and that it does not progress into systemic scleroderma.

◆ ❖ ◆

Joellen Brewster
Daughter Rachel, Morphea
Pennsylvania, USA

During the summer of 1999, we noticed that our daughter had a blotchy, purple-red rash all over the lower part of her left leg. After a trip to the local dermatologist, Rachel was given the diagnosis of dermatitis and some cortisone cream to apply to the area. This did nothing for the rash.

This rash did not seem to bother Rachel, so my husband and I assumed that, perhaps, it was some sort of allergic reaction as the dermatologist had suspected. My husband and I both have allergies and assumed that our daughter had inherited them. The dermatologist had suggested allergy testing when she got a little older, and we were going to follow up with that.

As the summer turned into fall, we noticed that Rachel started to experience some stiffness in her knee and, coincidentally (or so we thought at the time), it was in the left knee on the same leg as the rash. After trips to an orthopedic doctor (who diagnosed psoriatic rheumatoid arthritis) and a rheumatologist (who diagnosed pauciarticular rheumatoid arthritis), we were referred to a pediatric rheumatologist who thought it was scleroderma.

When I first heard the word scleroderma, I almost fell on the floor. The only form of scleroderma I knew about was the systemic kind, and I immediately thought my daughter was going to die. The doctor took a lot of time to explain morphea to us and subsequently confirmed his diagnosis with a skin biopsy.

Rachel is returning to the pediatric rheumatologist in the next few days and will start treatment. The morphea has also spread up the left side of her body, and she now has patches on her stomach, left shoulder blade, behind her left ear, and around her hairline at the nape of her neck.

I am so grateful there are websites like this where I can get information and get in contact with other people who are living with morphea, and particularly from parents coping with a child with morphea.

Update – May 2000

Rachel is currently on treatments, which she will take over the next six months with a gradual tapering off. She will continue on methotrexate for about eighteen months. The doctor said that after being off medication, we will look for any signs of progression of the illness and use more medication, if the illness continues to progress.

Rachel is also going to physical therapy this week to help with range of motion in her foot and leg affected by the morphea. She will also have some massage techniques on the plaques, or hardened areas of skin. My husband and I will learn these exercises and massage techniques so we can continue them when physical therapy is over.

Other than some puffiness in the face, caused by the prednisone, Rachel really has not had any side effects from the medicines. So far, so good!

Update – Early June 2001

Rachel is now off the prednisone and continues her weekly dose of methotrexate. However, the leg that has been affected is still significantly smaller than her other leg. The doctor has some concern over this, as do my husband and I.

She may have to have some special lifts (orthotics) for her shoes to make sure her walking is normal due to the size and length differences in the legs. She will be seeing an occupational therapist and physical therapist at her next doctor's visit in a couple of weeks. The doctor is considering an MRI to evaluate the depth to which the morphea has affected her leg, with respect to muscle and bone growth. I do not like the idea of an MRI because Rachel will have to be anesthetized to ensure she will lie still during the procedure, which is a lot to ask of a four year old! I know it has to be done if that is what is best for her, but I still do not like it!

Actually, I do not like any of it. I would rather cut off my right arm than have a sick child, but we cope as best as we can and always hope and pray for the best.

Update – Late June 2001

We saw the pediatric rheumatologist this week as well as the physical therapist. The physical therapist recommended a built-up heel for Rachel's shoe on the affected leg because it is about a half inch shorter than the other. This will help her walk more normally and prevent any problems a length difference can create.

The doctor has also decided to do the MRI within the next month. Based on the MRI, he can decide what type of medication will encourage her leg to grow. He thought he could possibly put her back on the prednisone or other immunosuppressant drugs to help her. He plans to consult with other physicians in Pittsburgh and New York City because they see more cases of this than he does.

So we are just waiting to have the MRI done and we will go from there. Just for a helpful hint to others: check with your insurance before your child has an MRI. If anesthesia is necessary to keep a child still, your insurance may require a letter from your doctor explaining why the anesthesia is medically necessary; otherwise, the anesthesia portion of the procedure may not be covered. Obviously, they have never had to keep a child still for longer than a minute or they would know!

Update – January 2002

Rachel had her MRI in October 2001, and the good news is the scleroderma only goes as deep as the fat; there is no involvement in the muscle and bone. We were very relieved and thankful for that news. We had another visit with the rheumatologist in January and learned that the growth difference between Rachel's upper thighs (the affected leg versus the healthy leg) is now only 1 cm., meaning her affected leg has actually grown!

She has grown three-quarters of an inch taller between October and January. I was so happy with this news, I could have cried. The areas on her affected leg have softened significantly and do not seem to be as deep. The skin is not as dry as it once was.

Things are going really well. Thanks to all the people who have emailed me. Take care, everyone, and God bless!

Joyce L. Priore
Daughter Cassi, Morphea
Rhode Island, USA

Shortly after I started a new position at a local casino, my older daughter, Lauren, told me that she had noticed bruises on her sister Cassi's chest when they were taking a bath. I carefully checked Cassi's bruises when she came into the living room. Cassi, age six, said that they did not hurt and that no one had hit her.

I watched her carefully for several days and the bruises did not change. When Lauren went to the pediatrician that week, I also had him check out Cassi. He seemed unconcerned, but said to check back with him after one week, if they remained unchanged.

I was still concerned, so I took her with me to a dermatologist's appointment I had that week. The dermatologist immediately suspected scleroderma and performed a biopsy of the largest bruise. The biopsy was positive for morphea. I went home and started to research everything I could find on the disease. I did not like what I found.

With no real promising information available, I went to talk with the dermatologist again. An autoimmune disease had to start from some type of irritant, I had surmised, so we spoke of her problem with processed meats. Meat had caused digestive problems for her since birth, but fresh game meats did not bother her. I put her back on a natural diet of fresh fruits, vegetables, and venison immediately.

Within three short weeks, the disease had completely stopped progressing. Slowly, the six or seven areas affected lost their odd coloring and now appear as slightly discolored spots (similar to that of a kid who refuses to wash behind his ears). The largest affected area has some deep collagen problems and has since torn as she has grown, but no new areas have surfaced. She is now almost sixteen and continues with her natural diet with a couple of fast-food burgers snuck in about once a month.

We believe that the steroids, dyes, antibiotics, etc., used in cattle and meat processing, are part of the problem for Cassi. We also live in a high incident area for the disease.

When Cassi was nine, a first-grade student at her school died of scleroderma; a man I grew up with died from the disease; another schoolmate of mine, who is now a hospital administrator, has a rapidly progressive form of the disease; and a Pequot Indian woman who worked with me to try to find the cause of Cassi's morphea also has had problems with scleroderma. These people all have lived within a five-mile radius of each other for most of their lives.

Cassi is thankful for each and every day that she is unaffected by a new outbreak of her disease, and we pray that a cure will be found for her and all the other people affected with morphea.

Kathy Gaither
Son B. J., Juvenile Scleroderma
California, USA

Kathy Gaither is the Founder and President of the Juvenile Scleroderma Network Inc., at www.jsdn.org, an organization that provides support and friendship to children who have Juvenile Scleroderma.

My son B. J. was no different from any other toddler until one day in preschool, the teacher reported to me that he was having difficulty cutting with the scissors and with finger painting. I started to notice shortly after that he was not as active as other children, and he was not able to use his hands like other children. B. J.'s right fingers were becoming a bit crooked. His pediatrician suspected it could possibly be arthritis and immediately sent us to a pediatric rheumatologist.

In December of 1995, the pediatric rheumatologist ordered a number of blood tests every two weeks. My son was so terrified of needles that it took my mom, another person, and me just to hold him down. It broke my heart to see him this way. After the first blood test came back, the pediatric rheumatologist was not sure what B. J. had. He mentioned it could be juvenile rheumatoid arthritis (JRA), lupus, or leukemia. I had to wait a month to find out what he had because the hospital kept losing his blood test.

Finally, when he was four years old, he was diagnosed with JRA and put on anti-inflammatories for pain and stiffness. He had a hard time getting in and out of a car or bed. There were times he would fall to the ground and could not walk because of the pain.

There was no improvement, so I decided to take him to another pediatric rheumatologist. This doctor agreed that B. J. had JRA, and put him on methotrexate. By this time, he had started missing a lot of school. He could not play a lot of outside activities with the kids his age.

After months of this treatment, B. J. still showed no improvement. On the right side of his arm, he developed light and dark skin pigmentation. The doctor thought it was fungus. B. J. started to lose his hair in the back. He no longer had prints on the bottoms of his feet, and his right leg was shorter than the left.

Because B. J. was so stiff and his skin was becoming tight, his doctor decided to send him to the rehabilitation unit at Children's Hospital. He had to have seven hours of physical therapy and occupational therapy for five weeks.

It was just a few days before he was to go into the hospital when I noticed he had a brown, shiny spot on his stomach. I called the doctor, who looked at B. J. as soon as he arrived. The doctor examined him and ordered some blood tests. In a couple of days, I heard the word "scleroderma" for the first time. When the doctor said this word, I thought, "sclero what?" I only received one pamphlet to read about this disease. It was mentioned to me that there is not much information about this disease, especially in children.

After I read just about everything on systemic scleroderma, I thought my son was going to die. Because I knew nothing about scleroderma, I thought there was only one type. I was wrong, because my son has linear scleroderma.

After all this time, we thought my son had JRA when he actually had juvenile scleroderma (JSD). I could not believe he was misdiagnosed all those months. To find out that there is no cure for scleroderma just broke my heart all over again.

I became depressed for a year. Then finally, in August of 1997, I decided to accept scleroderma into my vocabulary. I was not going to let the disease run us; we were going to run the disease. I started educating myself more on scleroderma and educating the schoolteachers about it.

After two years, in August of 1999, I realized there was not enough support for parents of children with JSD. I decided I was going to turn our negative experience with scleroderma into something positive for us and for other parents. That's when I founded the Juvenile Scleroderma Network (JSDN), which I run out of my home. I have found the best therapy for dealing with your own child's chronic illness is to participate in a support group of similar issues regarding children.

Now B. J. is nine years old, and JSD continues to progress throughout the right side of his body. He had hand surgery in January 2000 to help correct the deformity in his wrist and fingers. Of course, at times he gets really upset that he can't do what other kids his age can do.

My son is my inspiration, because I admire how he tries to live a life without limitations and frustrations, dealing with a disease every day. It takes a lot of courage to get up every morning to see what challenges will come his way. There are times I think he handles having JSD better than I do.

I truly believe there is a reason why JSD came into our lives: to help other families with children who have JSD until there is a cure. And beyond that cure, I will always be here to help others and learn from my son.

◆ ❖ ◆

Tammy Campbell
Daughter Davie, Linear Scleroderma
Michigan, USA

My beautiful, talented daughter was diagnosed with linear scleroderma at the age of fourteen. She had just won a ballet scholarship to Las Vegas University for two weeks in the summer. Davie had performed in the Nutcracker Ballet in December when she came down with a high fever and what the doctor called a sun fungus on her right arm.

The doctor gave Davie antibiotics and cream for her arm, and also said she had strep throat. Nothing was mentioned of her arm again until March 2001. She ran out of her cream and said it hurt if she did not use it.

I looked at her arm and there was a white line from the fingers to the shoulder. After approximately thirty doctors, she was diagnosed with scleroderma. She is now sixteen and can only straighten her arm to a ninety-degree angle. Thankfully, it did not spread to any other areas.

She is on medication, when I can get her to take it. She tried the UVA1 therapy at the University of Michigan, but to no avail.

Dr. Maureen Mayes has said Davie could be a candidate for skin grafts. We have to wait and see. If anyone has tried this, I would love some input. Davie continues her love for dance. She is also on the varsity pom-pom team at school.

Valerie
Son with Morphea
California, USA

We noticed that our son was developing a purplish rash on his left leg when he was about four years old. The doctor did not know what it was, but prescribed a steroid or cortisone cream, which had no effect.

As he grew, we noticed other patches on his back and side. When he was about eight years old, a doctor took a biopsy of the area on his leg and hip. He said that it was morphea and there was no known treatment.

Soon our son began to get bruised or dirty-looking patches on his face, and his teachers complained of poor hygiene. Of course, we let them know it was not dirt!

We have always asked for updated information whenever he has had a regular doctor's appointment. No one has ever mentioned any treatments. He saw a dermatologist recently who also gave us no hope.

Our son is sixteen now. The morphea has caused him much emotional pain, although he does not seem to have any motion restrictions or physical pain. One side of his face looks very gaunt and almost sunken in. He has a dark line and slight indentation going down the center of his forehead. Dark patches are on much of his face. One side of his chin is smaller than the other.

We are excited to see that there is information on the Internet where people pay attention to one another, and where we can find some help, hope, and support.

◆ ❖ ◆

CHAPTER 6

Localized Scleroderma
Linear and Morphea

*I believe in using the power of the
mind to make your dreams come true.*

— William "Bill" A. Miknius

Alex
Italy

I am a thirty-four-year-old woman, and I have been suffering from localized scleroderma for about twenty years.

The disease initially started with a very small mark on my right thigh that seemed to be a bruise. Then the lesion changed its appearance and extended along the entire leg. Meanwhile, a small mark also appeared on my face, which was almost certainly another manifestation of the same disease.

I went to see various specialists, almost all of whom agreed on the diagnosis and on the impossibility of an ad hoc therapy, explaining to me that the real cause of the disease is unknown, along with its treatment.

They suggested I try various treatments that have not been of much benefit apart from softening the skin.

I had a series of immunological tests performed (including antinuclear antibodies) to check if this was a systemic form of scleroderma. Fortunately, these tests were all negative.

Now, having read the information on www.sclero.org, I am no longer sure that these results completely rule out the more serious form of this disease. For the record, I also suffer from celiac disease.

Editorial note, revised in 2006: There was a widespread belief until quite recently that localized scleroderma (such as morphea or linear) could never progress to systemic disease. Recent research indicates that localized scleroderma can progress into systemic disease in about 0% to 2% of cases, depending on the study. Anticentromere antibodies may help to identify the subset of morphea or linear patients who may be at risk for progression. Also, about one-fourth of morphea or linear patients may develop one or two symptoms outside of skin involvement, including neurological involvement associated with linear scleroderma or Parry-Rombergs Syndrome.

◆ ❖ ◆

William "Bill" A. Miknius
Pennsylvania, USA

In 1975, when I was five years old, they said I was the fourth known case of localized scleroderma in a male in the United States. I have a deformed left foot and right hand. I have scleroderma plaques covering my left leg, stomach, chin, forehead, and lower back.

I have had so many different tests done and doctors from all over the world look at me and take pictures of me, I could write a book! There have been good times and bad times.

I am thirty-two years old now, and I have a beautiful wife and four beautiful children.

All I want to say is that life will go on. I think we should do what makes us happy: pray, fish, ride motorcycles, whatever—and remember there is always someone out there who is worse off than we are. I believe in using the power of the mind to help make dreams come true.

Anna
Poland

My story started nine years ago. On August 11, 1993, at the age of eighteen, I was admitted to the hospital because of arthritis in my big joints, which had developed over the prior six months. Based on the clinical picture as well as on some investigations, a diagnosis of juvenile rheumatoid arthritis (JRA) was made. I was transferred to the rheumatology ward for further investigation and specialist treatment because I was seriously ill.

On clinical examination, I was pale, my heart rate was high and my liver was enlarged. There was joint contraction at my elbows, limited movement in my shoulders and knees, and pain and functional limitation in my wrists and metatarsal joints. An erythrocyte sedimentation rate (ESR) test revealed increased inflammation, anemia, reduced iron levels, and erythrocytes in my urine. Immunological investigations showed the presence of LE cells as well as a high antinuclear antibody (ANA) titer. These findings led to a diagnosis of systemic lupus erythematosus (SLE).

During my stay in the hospital, I was found to have altered microcirculation with livedo reticularis as well as tight skin on my right lower limb, in particular, the dorsolateral part of my right foot. These abnormalities suggested another diagnosis: mixed connective tissue disease (MCTD). After three months of hospital care, I was generally well and was discharged with a specific treatment including steroids. I was advised to return for regular follow-ups at the rheumatology clinic.

This was the beginning of the difficulties in fully diagnosing my disease. At that time, I did not realize the severity of these diseases and where they can lead. I continued my existence, took my medication, and, at the same time, I was a witness to how one of these diseases was taking my father away.

The disease was destroying him slowly, as it involved his heart. Then one day he fell asleep and never woke up. His death was a horrible shock. I became an orphan, together with my brothers, including one who lived abroad. We had already lost our mother when we were small.

Five months later, the skin started to tighten over my right leg and arm. This prompted me to seek help at the hospital where I had been previously treated. Another diagnosis was made: an overlap syndrome of SLE and scleroderma.

After a month, as some specialist tests were unavailable in order to confirm the diagnosis, I was transferred to the dermatology clinic. The diagnosis this time was localized linear scleroderma and rheumatoid arthritis.

At this point, I wanted to know more about scleroderma. I suspected that it was a severe disease, and I wanted to understand it. In the hospital, I met three patients with scleroderma. They looked like mummies. One of them had short fingers and tight skin over her face, and it seemed to me that even pronouncing words caused her pain. I was very afraid that I was watching myself in the future and that this was what I should expect.

How does a young girl feel, looking at the long-term changes resulting from the disease with which she has just been diagnosed? Well, I felt very much afraid of dying, of dying too early, and of great suffering. I felt resentful that it had happened to me. All my plans for the future were black. I closed myself down and waited for what would happen next. I am not quite able to describe what I was really feeling, but I know that anyone who has not had this experience will not entirely understand what the patient is feeling.

In the hospital, one of the patients loaned me a book about scleroderma. After reading that book, I could not believe this was happening to me. I asked myself why, but I could not find an answer. I only knew that linear scleroderma is not so dangerous, that it involves the skin, but not the internal organs, and that it can only make a person handicapped.

Actually, I was not quite sure which form I was really suffering from and, therefore, I was hoping to have the less severe disease. The doctors were still uncertain whether I had overlap syndrome or severe linear scleroderma. I was transferred again, this time to an internal medicine and rheumatology ward. After two weeks, I was finally diagnosed with MCTD. As far as I could understand, it was neither severe linear scleroderma nor SLE. I was not sure which diagnosis had the worst prognosis, and I was desperate to know what to believe as different diagnoses had been made in different hospitals. Only now do I understand that differential diagnosis in the connective tissue disorders is not easy.

After being discharged from the hospital in 1994, I was really down. I did not know what to expect. My brother, who had been living with me, left the country. I was alone with my disease, which I hated and did not want to accept. Constant pain in my joints, as well as ever-increasing hardening of the skin of my leg and arm, were efficient reminders that I was ill. I did not believe I had any chance to have a normal life; the future did not exist for me. I stopped all treatment and started to drink alcohol; I did not care for anything. I drank and when my joint pain was worse, I took steroids. After some time, my leg appeared burned. There was muscular atrophy and the skin was extremely hard, in particular over my right leg. In order to forget, I drank even more. The summer was the worst season for me. I was condemned to sweat, wearing long trousers and long-sleeved shirts. Walking around the city and seeing smiling and normally dressed people, I felt sad I was not a part of them anymore. Alcohol became my best friend.

After two or three months, my rheumatic symptoms decreased, appearing only from time to time. I managed to get used to them. From 1994 to 1998, my life did not have any sense. I lived day by day and I was thinking of how to die. Then I realized I was pregnant—an event that restored my desire to live. I felt as if I had been born again. I was very happy but also worried for my unborn child because I had abandoned treatment for so long. Surprisingly, alcohol had not caused any particular changes in my body. My disease seemed to stop for a while, but not for long. I would never have thought that with this disease I would still be able to have a child. I very much wanted a girl. My disease was quiescent during pregnancy. I was feeling like a normal, healthy woman who was carrying a new life inside her. I realized I had given up too early and lost hope, which is so necessary for treatment. I did not give myself a chance for a normal life. I had been destroying myself.

It was my pregnancy that changed everything, and it was a beginning of my new life with a desire to fight against my disease. During nine months of pregnancy, I was taking care of my baby and myself, and everything was going very well. I did not let myself think something could go wrong; I just believed that my child would make me happy—that hope can make miracles. Finally, the day of delivery came and I gave a birth to a healthy girl. It was the happiest day in my entire life. Now I had somebody to live for.

On New Year's Eve, 1998, I met a man and we fell in love. He also has changed my life. Several months later, my disease started to upset me again and put me down. I could not get out of bed and needed hospital care. After two weeks I was discharged, but this time I decided to follow the treatment plan since there was someone who needed me. One year later we got married. My husband accepts me as I am. I realized that external appearance is not so important and what really counts is a family and love, without which life is hard, whether or not you are sick or healthy. Thanks to my husband, I have accepted myself.

In 2001, in the dermatology department, a diagnosis of a quiescent localized scleroderma of my right leg and arm was made; the treatment required only an organized lifestyle and careful skin care. I am currently undergoing a specialist's treatment for my rheumatic disturbances. In spite of many bad experiences, I am happy that my life has gained its sense of purpose again. I realized it is not worthwhile to give up. Even during the most difficult moments, it is necessary to fight and to believe that it will be better. If I had not believed, I would not be alive now. My daughter is now three and a half years old, and my husband and I are hoping to have another child. I now know that my disease is not hereditary and that a healthy mother can give a birth to a sick child, the same as a sick mother can have a healthy child.

Dora
Ontario, Canada

I was diagnosed with linear scleroderma (en coup de sabre) in Romania forty-one years ago. I feel I have to share with you my experience, mostly to give courage to the families with children diagnosed with scleroderma. Somehow, I feel it is my duty to tell you my story.

As often presented in the medical books, at age eleven, I had a violet stripe, which separated my forehead into two parts. It appeared quite suddenly, and my family and I went to see a dermatologist. The diagnosis of juvenile scleroderma shocked my family but, luckily, not me. I was just a kid then, a fourth-grade student, and I felt different because everybody told me how rare my disease was. Everybody kept telling me how lucky I was to have this particular form of the disease, and they were right. Meanwhile, I think I was grateful that it was not a difficult-to-bear disease as I was able to learn and play and to have quite a normal life.

For two months, I was hospitalized in Bucharest where the doctors were very kind to me, made me pictures, and treated me with medications. I will always remember one doctor. His name was Bolkonski. I had been reading Tolstoy's *War and Peace*, so I was excited to meet someone whose ancestors were so famous. As for my disease, the color of the stripe faded, but the skin was still thick and hard and adhered to my cranium.

My life continued like any child and continued like any teenager, except that I always had hair tangles on my forehead where the strip was. It still is very thin, hard and adhered.

I used to be a good student, and I entered the university. After finishing my studies at age twenty-three, I observed that the strip slowly became pink and I was losing hair. It was my first year as a country secondary school teacher in my hometown. I was again hospitalized for three months. My doctor gave me vasodilators, blood thinners, and chelation therapy. Because my blood tests were not the best at the beginning, the treatment was long, but not painful. Thank you for your help, Dr. Pantea, wherever you are!

It was only then I realized what sort of disease I have had. I will explain what I mean by "had" in the past tense.

From then on, I frantically read whatever I could find about scleroderma, and I felt quite puzzled that I did not feel anything strange, not even fatigue. I must confess I was scared to death that something could go wrong and how awfully wrong.

When I was about thirty-three years old, my collagen and antibodies blood tests became quite normal again, so I took only some herbal pills from France and a related unguent.

As I arrived in Canada almost five years ago, my then-future husband took me to Dr. Lee, a well-known rheumatologist in Toronto. Dr. Lee declared me both very lucky and cured from my juvenile scleroderma. That is why I used the word "had" in the past tense.

Deep, deep in my soul, I still fear a recurrence of any kind. How did I manage to live with scleroderma? Luckily, I managed to always keep myself busy by teaching and trying to have a family of my own in Romania, and by refusing to meditate too long about the scleroderma. Now I am busy with my new family, and I am continuing my studies. I try to enjoy life as I always have tried, and also give the world a smile and a kind word as often as possible.

Deep in my heart there is a feeling of guilt for the people who were not as lucky as me. I wish them all a lot of courage and trust in their selves as well as in their families and friends. I will always remember the words of an old and very nice lady I met in Greece: "Never give up!"

Please, my friends, my family, and all the people involved one way or another with scleroderma—you are also my family: "Never give up!"

Emma Walkinton
New Zealand

My linear scleroderma started on my left cheek at the age of four and by the time I was eight, that side of my face was quite deformed.

The growth of my left jawbones were affected; hence, the removal of teeth when I was sixteen in preparation for surgery. My mouth does not close as the lips cannot cover my protruding top jaw, and there is little saliva flow over these teeth.

From what I remember, the proposed surgery was to break my top jaw and make it fit my mouth without touching the skin that had been affected by the scleroderma. This skin is now quite soft.

This surgery, I presume, would also improve my bite. At the moment, my jaw does not meet and chewing is difficult.

Now the doctors seem to be reticent to cut into the scleroderma skin to puff out my cheek to make it look normal. My family and I are not critical of this or the five years on the waiting list, but at twenty-three, I would like something done.

I would love to hear from anyone who has linear scleroderma or had reconstructive facial surgery for it, or who is knowledgeable about such procedures.

Update – May 2002

My long-awaited facial surgery is scheduled for December.

◆ ❖ ◆

Amber
Utah, USA

My story with morphea started two years ago. I went to a tanning salon in February of 2000 and got horribly burned on my thighs and buttocks. It was so bad that it looked as if I had been caned. I figured it was just a burn and would go away. The skin on the back of my left upper thigh never got better, and it looked like a bruise. I paid no attention to it until November when it began to spread down my thigh.

I went to the dermatologist and he quickly diagnosed it as morphea. He told me it was related to scleroderma and would go away on its own without any intervention. Unfortunately, I watch the *Lifetime* TV show frequently, so I knew about systemic scleroderma, and I was shocked and scared. He reassured me that although it is related, it would never turn systemic. After a couple more visits with him, I was convinced he was no expert on the matter and sought out another doctor as the morphea continued to spread.

The doctor I now see has treated hundreds of patients with morphea and has claimed to see some patients' morphea turn systemic. This scares me to death because recently I have noticed several odd things going on.

In early February 2002, I began to have sharp, shooting pains that originate in my lower back and go down into my legs. My lower back was horribly sore, and it was difficult to sleep at night. In addition to the shooting pain, my muscles were sore in the back and sides of my legs.

About two weeks later, I noticed a tremendous and visible decrease in the amount of cellulite on the backs of my thighs, despite no change in my eating or exercise habits. I attributed this to skin thickening. I also noticed a burning sensation in the backs of my legs.

To date, the back of my right leg is still sore. The skin on my upper arms is not horribly sore, just a little sore to the touch. I have also begun to have pains in my ankles and forearms that seem to be in the bone. My legs, fingers, and feet often itch. And I am terribly tired all the time.

I called my dermatologist today to inform him of these changes. He wants me to come in next Monday and is very concerned. I wonder if I am the only person with morphea experiencing these other things. I also wonder if anyone with progressive systemic sclerosis started out with a diagnosis of morphea.

◆ ❖ ◆

Anita
Washington, USA

I want to share my story with scleroderma, which spans nearly eighteen years now. After a traumatic experience in my first year of college, during which I saw a dear friend drown, and another drown trying to rescue him, I returned home with a small, white patch on my back.

The patch did not itch and slowly grew to about an inch long over the course of a year. Normally blessed with excellent skin, I truly believed it would get better and that the discoloration would go away. It did not. It grew harder and would mildly itch. I was fairly careless and carefree at that time, so when a skin specialist diagnosed me with scleroderma, I did not even blink.

I was given strong ointments that greatly helped to soften the area; however, a while later I realized that the ointment had a very high steroid content. I noticed the effect the steroids were having on me during that time. I stopped the treatment when only a small patch of hard skin remained.

Since then, I have been on homeopathy. And while stressful factors have caused the patch to become inflamed occasionally, I generally remain in good health.

Betty Jones
Texas, USA

In June of 1999, after getting a tan at the beach, I noticed a little white spot that was three inches directly above my belly button. I thought I was peeling from too much sun.

By October, I had these white spots all over my stomach. Over the next eight months, three different doctors all misdiagnosed me with tinea versicolor, which is a type of fungus.

By February 2001, the spots were on my stomach, the top of my thighs, and on my back. There were also brown, scaly patches on the underside of my upper arms.

I went to a dermatologist, who did an incision biopsy and diagnosed me with localized scleroderma (morphea). It is cutaneous morphea; meaning, it is only on the skin. He told me the cause is unknown, there is no known cure, and it is not contagious. He told me it is unlikely that it would turn into anything worse, and it would probably go away in a few years.

I immediately got on the Internet and decided to make an appointment with a rheumatologist. I want to make sure that nothing internal is being affected. And I also want to find out if there is any medication to make these spots go away.

Luckily, I am pretty fair-skinned, so the spots are only noticeable when I get tan.

Dienne Mickey
Ohio, USA

At age ten, I developed a rash on my leg that never went away and would not respond to any treatment. Subsequently, I was diagnosed at age fifteen with morphea scleroderma.

I knew nothing about the disease and went on with my life thinking I had a skin disease. I have the neck ring, and everyone thought I had a dirty neck. I also have the discoloration on my forearms and across my lower back.

Since my initial diagnosis, I have had four pregnancies. One was a miscarriage and my last two were premature. I had four spontaneous pneumothoraxes (collapsed lung) in three months and severe migraines, two of which resulted in stroke-like symptoms.

I finally saw a rheumatologist about six years ago who told me I had Raynaud's phenomenon and telangiectases (spider veins) on my hands. Blood work was ordered, but I was getting a divorce and as soon as the divorce was final, I lost my health insurance, so I never went back to the doctor.

These last few months, I have had asthma attacks or tightening in my chest, and heart palpitations. I freeze in air-conditioning, and I have just recently developed lesions on my torso. In just one week the lesions went from size two to size twenty-three, with all but one of them being symmetrical.

I have also been complaining of joint pain, but my blood work shows no arthritis. I am tired, but do not suffer from diabetes or hypothyroidism (which runs in my family). Since the lesions have appeared, my hips hurt constantly.

I am looking for someone else who may have the same symptoms, as this disease affects us all differently. I am finally going to a rheumatologist at the Cleveland Clinic where they say they have several scleroderma patients, so they are familiar with it. Different doctors have told me that because my test results come back normal, it must be in my head! I know: "Been there, done that!"

Update – February 2002

I designed the logo for the International Scleroderma Network as the result of a class project I did while attending Virginia Marti College of Art and Design in Lakewood, Ohio. I earned my Associates Degree in Graphic Design in the spring of 2002.

I have morphea with possible CREST. I have a cousin with diffuse scleroderma, and my only sister has lupus. This is why scleroderma awareness is a high priority for me. I feel that the more people and doctors know about this rare and baffling disease, the closer we come to finding its causes and its cure.

We all need people who understand what we are going through. Thank you for the opportunity to share my story.

Jenny Meade
Florida, USA

It started like a purple bruise that never healed. Then the itching began along with noticeable loss of pigmentation. I kept ignoring the symptoms thinking it was a sunspot or something of that nature. When my leg became swollen, I could not ignore it anymore.

I went to several doctors. I was told it was a fungus and, further, that it was clearly all in my head. I went to a dermatologist who told me it was vitiligo. Another said it was lichen sclerosus. Eight months into the disease, I was finally referred to a rheumatologist who has recently diagnosed me with morphea. I have started taking medication for it, but it is really too early to see any signs of improvement. I hope it works.

Update – May 2001

Life with morphea is harsh. I have experienced more difficulty with what should be easy tasks. I continuously find myself opening a two-liter bottle or a milk jug with my teeth. My hands are no longer able to close into a fist position. I cannot straighten my left leg or my left arm. I wear sandals most of the time because my foot is in such bad shape.

I hate this disease and have trouble understanding how or why this is happening to me. I miss the person I was and hate the person I have become. I have hope that one day I will be able to wear shorts and run alongside my son without having to worry about what people think when they look at me.

Now I am on medication recommended by a doctor from the University of South Florida Health Sciences Center. I hope that it will work for me. I am twenty-three and terrified that I am limited to what I do and how I do things. I think about my future and find more and more things that I have not done and probably will not do. I would love to go back to school, but worry about having to write papers, anticipating the pain that my hands would experience.

Although I am finding this to be the most terrifying and terrible time in my life, even more so than when I miscarried, I am finding a little bit of self-acceptance. This new treatment has reduced some of my symptoms and given me hope. As I see or feel any improvement, I believe my 'self' will start returning.

◆ ❖ ◆

Julie L. Thompson
Indiana, USA

I am now thirty-two years old and have had morphea for almost twenty years. Unfortunately, it has not stopped and it has taken over a lot of my body: my stomach, back, right arm, both legs, right hand, both feet, and neck.

The morphea is mostly dark in color with some being white and plaque-like. I was on medication for almost ten years with little to no effect. When I started having children, I had to stop the medicine.

I have also tried PUVA light treatments, but to no avail. I now receive cortisone shots into the lesions every time a new lesion appears, which is hard to tell because they are so widespread.

I am done having children now and am looking for something else to try. I am interested in experimental treatments aside from just using makeup to minimize the existing scars. I feel very emotional about this at times, but I am grateful that, so far, I do not have any internal problems.

Krysten Fox
Massachusetts, USA

I remember sitting on my dad's lap when I was five, and he called my mother into the room to look at my left leg where the skin had become very tight and oddly textured.

A trip to my pediatrician left my parents in search of a second opinion, because there was no way that what was happening to me was simply the result of growing too fast. It is a little hard to remember all the details considering I was only five years old. Regardless, I was diagnosed with scleroderma.

I was told it was a disease that was very rare in elderly people and even more so in children. I also remember something about calcium and my lack of drinking enough milk.

My leg continued to become tighter and discolored. I remember a lot of hospital visits and one story about a girl, a few years older than me, who had it under her armpit area. Unfortunately for her, it was spreading pretty fast.

Even though I was unfortunate enough to get scleroderma, I found it hard to feel too bad about it. I knew from the beginning it could have been a lot worse. I do not remember being in much pain, and I have always lived an athletic, tomboy lifestyle.

The discoloration and texture traveled the length of my inner left leg, which is a quarter of an inch skinnier than my right. My knee is very thin and pretty much just bone. I have not been inhibited in any way. I have played soccer for the last twelve years and I was certainly considered one of the top athletes of my grade.

As far as I am concerned, the worst part of living with scleroderma was the awful tasting medicine I had to take when I was five. I have had to master the art of disguise and avoid wearing shorts. I am still not comfortable with the scar, but I have been free of scleroderma symptoms for quite some time. I know that I am a lucky one. It could have been a lot worse.

◆ ❖ ◆

Linda
Norway

I am a seventeen-year-old girl, and I just received the diagnosis of morphea. I have five big spots and two small ones. I have a cream from the doctor, and I hope it will help me! But he is not sure it will. I wonder if there are other methods of treatment.

I will do what I can to get the spots to go away or to prevent any new ones. I need all the help I can get.

Update – February 2002

I have four new spots. The doctor told me the skin condition would burn out after one to two years. I have had morphea for three years and although the new spots are getting worse, the old spots are really better.

I wonder when this will stop. Last year I went to Spain for a holiday, and the spots became much better. I think it is the sun that helped it a lot.

I do not think this is too bad with the new spots, but it is not funny when you can see that your skin looks worse and worse. I will not get depressed because of this. The emails of support I have received have helped me a lot!

Pamela Ward
California, USA

About ten years ago, my problem started with what I thought was a bruise about the size of a dime under my arm. At first I was told it was a fungus and given cream to treat it, but it did not work. The purplish spot began to get bigger, turning white in the middle. I went to several doctors, one of whom simply said it might be scleroderma and sent me on my way. I was horrified! I thought for sure I was going to die!

Then I found a dermatologist who did a biopsy and said it was morphea. She explained that it is caused by a buildup of collagen under the surface of the skin, which causes discoloration and hardening of the skin. She also told me that morphea stays at the surface of the skin and does not affect the organs or cause death. She said that usually morphea would lighten and sometimes even disappear in a couple of years.

She started injecting steroids into the hardened area to soften it. Once the spot was softened, she tried to get rid of the dark color. First, we used a roll-on preparation, but that did not work. Next, we tried the patches, but they only irritated my skin, making it red and very painful. We finally gave up and agreed to let nature take its course, hoping the discolored area would indeed disappear in a couple of years.

Now, ten years later, I have an enormous bruise-like thing under my arm that has also spread near my right breast. Another patch stretches about six inches across my lower back. I jokingly refer to this as my "Catalina scar." In case you are unfamiliar with it, Catalina is an island off the coast of Southern California. Recently, I have noticed the entire underside of my right arm is starting to discolor. Other than the disturbing appearance, the only thing I am bothered with is incessant itching.

I was hoping that after ten years someone might have found a cure or at least a way to stop the discoloration. I am not finding anything.

◆ ❖ ◆

Reza Gorjian
Son of Father with Morphea Scleroderma
Iran

I am writing from Iran. My father has had morphea scleroderma since 1990. The morphea patch appeared on his stomach and was about the size of a hand.

He went to a doctor in 1990, and the doctor gave him one thousand vitamin E tablets to fight the disease. Before going to the doctor, his skin was hard. After using the tablets, his skin became softer and the color started to return to the usual color. Then it stopped.

We thought that it was cured, but in 2001, it started up again as small spots on the other side of his stomach. Please tell me what can we do?

The doctor that we went to in 1990 is now dead, and the doctors in Iran do not have much information about this kind of disease. Please help me. I am worried about his health. Thanks.

Stephanie Goens
Florida, USA

In the year 2000, I finally received a diagnosis of localized morphea. I have bruise-like patches all over the trunk of my body. The spots grow under my breast, on my side, stomach, back, and part of my arm. It has confined itself to the left side of my body.

My doctor, at the time, told me not to worry, but at the same time said there is no cure. I think it is affecting my joints. I feel like I have arthritis at twenty-five years old.

Susan Shirley Allen
Australia

I am a thirty-eight year old woman living in South Australia, where there is a high incidence of morphea.

I suspect I have had a localized form of this, on and off, on the lower front shin of one leg for ten years. It may have started when I was heavily pregnant and I knocked my leg. It took eighteen months to resolve, and I felt feverish and unwell. It felt ten times worse than a bruised, raw feeling.

A dermatologist diagnosed morphea after a biopsy, although at first she thought it was erythema nodosum (another skin condition). Last year, I was wearing new hiking boots, which rubbed a spot on my ankle. The morphea became active again, and it went deep into my inner ankle.

I have been passed around among dermatologists and rheumatologists who now say I am developing rheumatoid arthritis in my right ankle and right hand. I feel these knocks and bruises, now turning into something more sinister, are related. I felt so unwell and feverish that I was wondering if it was hormonal, so I stopped taking the contraceptive pill three months ago. The nodule has gotten smaller and is spontaneously resolving. However, I am left with a deep ache in the ankle and in three fingers on my right hand.

I am finding it very hard to get anybody to listen to my thoughts and feelings, which I think are substantiated. Is there any evidence or information that morphea and arthritis are linked?

I feel this is more deep-seated than a dermatologist can handle. I am hoping to work with a professional and present them with any thoughts, feelings, and facts on the matter.

I feel for all of you and wonder if it took you as long to be diagnosed as it did for me.

◆ ❖ ◆

Tonya Raines
North Carolina, USA

I am thirty and was diagnosed with morphea when I was sixteen or seventeen. I originally went to the doctor because I had noticed a white, waxy lump on the back of my thigh. It did not hurt or itch, but my mom worried about it.

The general practitioner (GP) did not know what to make of it, so I was referred to a dermatologist. After a biopsy, I was told I had morphea. The doctor handed me a medical book and said he had only seen one other person with it before. He said the cause was unknown and there was nothing to be done about it. It was not life threatening and did not involve internal organs. I left his office unhappy, but my mom was thrilled I did not have cancer.

During the next few years, I noticed more and more spots. I could tell they were morphea, too, but they were different than the original white, waxy lump on my thigh. They had no white center. These were brown spots that sunk below the level of my skin. The worst thing is that they look like bruises from a distance, and several well-meaning but ignorant friends and family members have questioned whether or not I am a victim of domestic violence. This is completely unfair to my husband, who is very understanding! For this reason, I will not wear anything that shows my back, which is where most of the spots are located.

When I was twenty-eight, I went to another dermatologist at a university hospital here in North Carolina. After another biopsy and negative results for Lyme disease, I was again told it was morphea and given hydrocortisone cream for any new spots. They said it will not prevent the scarring, but it may cause it to burn out more quickly so the spots will be smaller. I haven't found any new or active spots in years.

After some Internet research, I realize that I am indeed one of the lucky ones (so far) and have not had any complications. It does make me feel a little less weird to know I am not alone. I have avoided the sun like the plague since my initial diagnosis, and I wonder whether tanning would help to hide the brown spots, or if it would only make them darker or worse, bring on another attack?

◆ ❖ ◆

PART 3

Autoimmune and Overlap

CHAPTER 7

Autoimmune Stories

I have learned that you can fight pulmonary fibrosis!.
— Bob Morris

Introduction
by Shelley L. Ensz

Shelley Ensz is Founder and President of the International Scleroderma Network.

Autoimmune illnesses like scleroderma often take many years to be properly diagnosed. This chapter features stories about difficult, delayed or revised diagnoses.

In the early stages of illness, when symptoms are often rather non-specific, it is easy to become focused on trying to achieve a diagnosis. It is common to think that having a proper diagnosis is critical to receiving proper treatment, and many of us find it hard to believe assurances that it is only important to have our symptoms properly treated.

It can quickly become a battle for self-esteem, as we seek to reassure ourselves, as well as our family, friends, doctors, employers, and disability examiners, that there is a real illness. We may begin to question whether we are at fault, perhaps thinking that doctors no longer take us seriously. Frequently, we interpret the lack of firm answers to mean that the doctors secretly suspect it is "all in our heads."

The stress of the illness and uncertainty about diagnosis may lead to anxiety or depression, and it may precipitate a questionable round of further medical consultations that often only adds to the confusion. Many of us turn to friends, coworkers, magazines, or even the Internet in search of answers. Sometimes we unearth the key to our diagnosis through a casual conversation, or through an exhausting search through medical volumes or websites. However, sometimes we may only succeed in stirring up the already murky diagnostic waters.

The truth is, when it comes to complex illnesses, there is often very little that can be done to hasten a diagnosis, no matter how eager and knowledgeable the patient, the caregiver, or the medical team.

Diagnosis of autoimmune and connective tissue diseases can take years, decades, and sometimes even a lifetime, with many diagnoses being made only in the last stages or by autopsy. It is common to have several symptoms of autoimmune (or other) diseases without ever developing classic symptoms of full-blown disease that lead to a definitive diagnosis.

Some of us have overlapping symptoms of multiple autoimmune diseases. This can lead to a never-ending cycle of new, different, discarded and revised diagnoses as our merry-go-round of symptoms changes over time.

We try to ease the confusion and despair of dealing with a difficult diagnosis by sharing our stories. In our stories there is a common thread that binds and comforts us by knowing others have also experienced a misguided diagnosis, a sad chain of events that caused needless suffering, doctors who knew little about scleroderma or other autoimmune diseases, or a confounding battery of tests.

We also gain strength from hearing about the persistence of those who knew something was wrong and didn't give up on the often long and troubling search for an accurate diagnosis.

These are the voices of support and the footprints we leave so the road for others will be less stressful. We welcome everyone with scleroderma or related illnesses or symptoms into our ISN support community, so that nobody needs to suffer alone or in silence.

Maureen "Buggzy"
Australia

I am a forty-six-year-old mother of three children, and I have two grandchildren. This might seem like a tirade, but I am anxious to know if anyone has had a similar experience. I have been diagnosed with fibromyalgia, ulcerative esophagitis, Gilbert's syndrome, diverticulitis, peripheral neuritis, and trigeminal neuralgia. I lost all taste sensation for about eight months, at one stage, but all that showed up in pathology was an elevated erythrocyte sedimentation rate (ESR).

When I was ten, I got this huge, black blood blister on the roof of my mouth, which stayed for years. I had it X rayed and they put it down as a mucous cyst, stating that it was highly unusual! Over the years, I have had blood blisters, the size of grapes, in my mouth. The doctors are mystified by it! I have also had blood blisters on my thighs, stomach, and chest as well as petechiae.

I have had surgeries for dislocated joints, a hernia, and removal of my gallbladder and tonsils. I have had a nephrectomy because of kidney cancer, and sutures to hold my pregnancies. I lost my first two babies preterm and all my kids were premature. My antinuclear antibodies (ANA) ranged between 1:40 to 1:640, and I have always had abnormal liver function tests as well as elevated serum ACE and ESR levels.

The only reason I have listed everything is in the hope that one of you may have had similar experiences. I know it sounds like a hypochondriac's diary, but I am really desperate to get some answers or to hear from others who are in the same boat as me.

Update

Since my first letter in 1999, I have had many unnamed illnesses. I am just getting over my third attack of trigeminal neuralgia. It is the most excruciating thing I have had to deal with. It lasted over a month this time and gradually subsided. My blood screens for this period were way off the chart. They showed extreme inflammation in my body. The doctor did not tell me the levels, but I had to go back for repeat tests. My hair was falling out by the truckload. I don't have any bald patches, just overall hair loss.

In May 2001, I developed three blisters the size of hardboiled eggs on my stomach. I foolishly burst them and copious amounts of fluid came out. The lesion had three points of hemorrhage on the surface, and it deteriorated into a severe ulcer. I had skin biopsies. Nobody offered a diagnosis. Nobody had any idea. Nobody had seen anything like it. Possibilities thrown at me included a burn and a white-tailed spider bite.

The biopsies simply showed ulceration. Eleven weeks later with fresh dressings every second day, none of us is wiser, except that I have a huge, ugly scar.

At the same time this was happening, my left knee started dislocating again for no reason, and my problems with endometriosis began. I felt bamboozled by all these things. My serum iron levels were very low, but the doctor suggested that this could have been from the loss of all the fluid through the ulcer on my stomach.

My fibromyalgia has been really bad over the last twelve months, and I find I have to sleep often. The trigeminal neuralgia caused my blood tests to be extremely abnormal. Over the last two years, I have had two hysteroscopies for endometritis (not endometriosis). It seems that instead of being 2 cm., my endometrium is 14 cm.—all due to inflammation.

My gynecologist just wants to wait and see if it sorts itself out. Of interest is that they have found I have an abnormal Alpha-1 Antitrypsin (A1A) gene, supposedly passed down through my Danish heritage. Since my last update, I have also had another liver biopsy, which showed inflammation, but no scarring. I have long ago given up trying to find what is wrong with me.

John Brophy
Connecticut, USA

I am sixty-one years old and currently collect disability. In late 1996, when I lived in Florida, I noticed overall swelling one day while I was driving to the golf course. The swelling persisted, so I saw an internist, who prescribed diuretics.

After two months of persistent swelling, my regular doctor sent me to a dermatologist who finally diagnosed me with eosinophilic fasciitis (EF) and treated me with steroids. The medication was not any help, even though I had all of the side effects.

Then he tried PUVA phototherapy with high doses of steroids. The swelling went away, but my skin became hard on parts of my legs, arms, and shoulders.

I still am addicted to sleeping pills, which are necessary to counteract the stimulating effects of the steroids. I came to the conclusion that the dermatologist was too reliant on steroids, so I went to a rheumatologist. He told me that I have a scleroderma-like condition. He tried every drug or intravenous treatment that could possibly help me, including chemotherapy, but to no avail.

I was part of a scleroderma clinical trial at the University of Connecticut Health Center with Dr. Naomi Rothfield and her fine staff, but it did not help. Next, I may join the new experiment in animal bovine collagen. I also went to Dr. Joseph Korn in Boston for his opinion. He thinks that I have eosinophilic fasciitis.

My current physical condition involves knee contractures that prevent me from walking, very tight skin in the leg area, and mild arm and hand tightness. I can type and wheel myself around in my wheelchair. I do not have any facial involvement.

Fatigue is the most difficult symptom, along with addiction to sleeping pills. I can only work for a couple of hours. Obviously, I cannot golf anymore, and restricted activity is the order of the day.

The doctors tried what is called "progressive casting" of my legs. During the second week of immobility, I developed a serious sore on my leg. The casts were taken off, and my legs are still not back in condition for casting again.

I am told that knee contractures are relatively rare in scleroderma. I seem to have the reverse of normal conditions; that is, more leg involvement and less skin tightness in the face and hands. I have no skin tightening in my fingers, except that they are very cold.

That is my story. I may need a new doctor, only because Boston is too far away for me. Perhaps there is a treatment center in Manhattan? Fortunately, I have a driver, plus a wheelchair in the trunk of the car.

Yvonne Frasure
Kentucky, USA

So far I have been diagnosed with fibromyalgia and Raynaud's phenomenon. In addition, two doctors are leaning toward a diagnosis of scleroderma, but I am not sure which type. One doctor believes I am developing CREST Syndrome.

I went for about two months throwing up everything I ate and although I would not feel like eating for a few days, I did not lose weight. I have a lot of pain throughout my muscles and around the joints for a few days at a time. My ANA is 1:1280.

Off and on, I either wheeze or have a burning sensation in the bottom of my lungs. If I exercise really hard, I have a bloody taste for about an hour afterward.

I have lapses of extreme exhaustion; I can fall asleep while typing. Then I can go for a long period and be fine. I feel like I am just imagining the bad days.

I am having trouble dealing with this because I have always been strong, with good endurance and able to concentrate. Now I feel like a whining hypochondriac. I am on three stomach medications and a calcium channel blocker.

Update – April 2002

As everyone does, I went from doctor to doctor, and I was seeing an internist up until last fall. She had sent for my blood tests from the rheumatologist and some information was missing. We did not retest and based on the information she had, along with my symptoms, I was diagnosed with CREST syndrome and fibromyalgia.

I am not sure about the progression of CREST. I have had this disease for at least four years, probably longer when I think back over the years at the symptoms I have had.

Anyway, I no longer go to the doctor because I simply cannot afford it. I cannot get insurance so everything is out-of-pocket, which can get very expensive. I am a senior in college at the ripe old age of thirty-four and still have a couple of years to go. Sometimes I wonder if I will make it. I plan to teach eventually.

My daily routine is to ignore whatever I feel and take care of my family. Sometimes it seems to be more of a chore than I can bear. My hands stay red and swollen, except when the Raynaud's phenomenon is running rampant with its red, white, and blue.

I have episodes of pain that occur with spontaneous bruising. I am not at all clear what that is. The fibromyalgia never completely lets up. The pain is constant: twenty-four/seven.

My hands and feet are shiny and stiff. I have esophageal dysmotility, telangiectasia, Raynaud's phenomenon, and apparently, sclerodactyly. These are four out of the five criteria for CREST. I have to admit, over the past few months, I have done considerably better (at least up until the past two weeks). Only time will tell. I believe in miracles—and I am waiting for mine.

Sherry Young
Arkansas, USA

I will be thirty years old in April. All my life, I was a thin, active, and popular girl. After the birth of my second child in 1995, I began to gain weight, ballooning up to two hundred and forty pounds within a year. I developed pneumonia on May 1, 1998, and after a chest X ray, I was told to see my doctor immediately.

My doctor informed me that I had a very large tumor on my thyroid. After a month of tests, the decision was made to operate. I was sent to a thoracic surgeon who scheduled me for surgery two days later. My entire sternum had to be opened to get this thing. When I woke up, he told me he had remove three-quarters of my thyroid and that I would have thyroid problems for life.

Let us fast-forward to 2001. My doctor took me off of thyroid medication in January because the dose caused hyperthyroidism. Nobody really knows how one-quarter of a thyroid can produce so many hormones on its own. One night in March, I was at work when, about 2 A.M., my pants suddenly felt tight. I went in the bathroom, pulled them down and was shocked to see my legs swollen to twice their normal size.

I told my boss I was going to the emergency room and called my boyfriend (now husband) to come get me. In the emergency room, the doctor on duty thought I had a blood clot and started me on injections and blood thinners until I could have a venous angioscopy three days later. That test showed nothing. My doctor then decided I had probably pulled a muscle in my back so he put me on steroids, which made my skin clearer, but did not do anything else. My left leg was tingly as if it had fallen asleep and had not woken up.

I continued working a very physically demanding job in a rice mill. As time went on, I began to be in constant pain. My feet would hurt, but it hurt worse to massage them. I could not even shave some parts of my legs, because they hurt too badly. I was falling apart, but being a divorced mother of two, I pressed on. My entire body hurt all the time. I became angry and irritable. My children were sometimes afraid to talk to me. My boyfriend was very supportive and together with my loving grandmother, they convinced me to see a local orthopedist.

He ran every test imaginable from bone scans to an MRI, blood work, and an EMG (a neuromuscular test) from which it took me a week to recover. Everything was negative. I became depressed and started thinking it was all in my head.

My family doctor sent me to a rheumatologist who finally diagnosed fibromyalgia. I was relieved to have a name for my problem. Although my family doctor had taken me off work on short-term disability two months earlier, the rheumatologist released me to go back full time with no restrictions.

He said fibromyalgia is just pain and if I could not handle my job, I should quit. After discussing this with my kids and fiancé, I went to my boss. We both agreed it would be better for me to resign than to get fired for not being able to do my job.

I still have a lot of problems including chronic pain, exhaustion, and inability to sleep. I have irritable bowel syndrome (IBS), headaches, and my leg is still asleep. I know that with time I will improve. I go back to my doctor soon, and due to what I have learned about fibromyalgia and thyroid problems, I am going to request some more tests.

Both sides of my family have a history of various autoimmune diseases, including my Aunt Cindy, whose story is also in this book.

I hope one day to lead a normal life, a life free of pain, with the energy to play with my children. For now, I will take one day at a time, counting on my faith to get me through.

Update – March 2002

My fiancé and I married on January 26th! I saw my family doctor last week. He did another thyroid study. My thyroid-stimulating hormone (TSH) was 1.77 and T was .71. He says both of these are normal and I should not worry. I have decided to refer myself to an endocrinologist.

My doctor also sent me to see a local cardiologist/pulmonologist (CP) for evaluation. He did not seem to be concerned about my leg swelling. He thinks it is probably hormonal, because I have a history of endometriosis and uterine fibroids. He referred me back to my gynecologist for that.

The CP scheduled me for a sleep study this month. He thinks I may have restless leg syndrome (RLS). My husband says I frequently stop breathing and gasp for air in my sleep. The CP doubts I have sleep apnea, because I do not have a lot of fat on my neck. He looked in my nose and noticed several polyps, which could be affecting my ability to breathe while I sleep. He recommended removal of the polyps.

Update – April 2002

I got the results of my sleep study today. The doctor said there were no significant findings, but he made the diagnosis of restless leg syndrome (RLS) because he said I fit the diagnostic criteria.

I showed the doctor my hands, which were a purple, mottled color. He asked me to remove my shoes and socks. I had purple, mottled toes! He quickly said, "Young lady, you have Raynaud's." He prescribed a medication for the RLS and gave me some tips for avoiding Raynaud's phenomenon flares. He told me to keep gloves in my purse and wear them if I go down the meat aisle at the supermarket. He also suggested oven mitts when retrieving things from the freezer.

I will see him again in two weeks. I also made an appointment in May with an endocrinologist to check my thyroid. It is going to take some getting used to, but I have learned to adapt to some new symptom on a seemingly weekly basis. Maybe I am back on the road to better health!

Tina Gibson
Tennessee, USA

I have systemic scleroderma. About twelve years ago and prior to being diagnosed, I was diagnosed with interstitial cystitis (IC).

Interstitial cystitis is a chronic inflammation condition of the bladder that can destroy the lining of the bladder and cause it to harden and shrink. The symptoms are frequent urination, pain, and pressure.

Unlike common cystitis, interstitial cystitis does not respond to conventional antibiotic therapy, and it is probably not caused by infection. There is no cure and after many different treatments, my bladder was removed in 1992.

Two to three years later, I developed muscle and joint pain, hypertension, Hashimoto's thyroiditis, arm numbness, and confusion. After seeing many doctors, including rheumatologists, I was diagnosed with systemic scleroderma. Therefore, I am interested in the relationship between interstitial cystitis and scleroderma. Thanks for your support.

-

Bob Morris
Pennsylvania, USA

June 8, 2000, was one of the low points of my life. I had just been diagnosed with pulmonary fibrosis, and tears coursed down my cheeks as I left my doctor's office. All I could think was how short my life would be, of all the things I still wanted to do, and of all the friends and relatives I would miss. I was wallowing in self-pity.

The next few months were filled with myriad visits to various specialists for MRIs, lung biopsies, X rays, and more. Despite the strong advice of all the experts about the importance of beginning treatment as soon as possible, I was not given any medication.

After I regained a bit of my equilibrium, my sister (who is a computer guru) and I began an intensive search on the Internet to learn as much as possible about pulmonary fibrosis and any promising medications. At first, we zeroed in on a drug that appeared quite promising, but we later learned that clinical trials of the drug had been disappointing.

Ultimately, I came across an article about an Austrian doctor who had conducted some very promising phase one clinical trials of interferon gamma and prednisone. In September 2000, I learned that additional wide-scale testing was starting in the United States. However, the trials were being done on a double-blind basis; meaning that even if I was qualified to participate in the trial, I could still end up taking a placebo rather than the actual drug! I elected to go off protocol, taking exactly the prescribed medication used in the study.

We shopped around for an inexpensive source of the interferon. My sister even went to Mexico to locate a supplier. The least expensive supplier we could find was one thousand dollars per week! At the time, no one would reimburse me for this horrendous expense but, as I saw it, I either take it or die. I was forced to sell some assets and I assumed a large debt, but it turned out to be worth every penny I spent. Now there is a chance that health insurance will start paying for this treatment.

In August 2000, I purchased an inexpensive oximeter to measure my blood oxygen saturation. Now able to monitor my pulmonary performance after commencing the treatment injections administered by my wife, there was a marked improvement in my condition. Since that time, my condition has stabilized and remained more or less unchanged for about a year.

During the past year, I have found I can participate in many activities without the use of supplemental oxygen. For instance, I can canoe, fly fish, travel by plane, hike on level ground, and dig clams. With four liters per minute of supplemental oxygen, I can bike, hike the Appalachian Trail, exercise in the gym, and generally do modestly strenuous activities. I also learned that working in cold weather uses much more oxygen than working in warm weather.

Altitude has a strong bearing on blood oxygen saturation. For every one-thousand foot increase in elevation, oxygen saturation decreases by about one percent. Oxygen saturation, as measured in the finger, does not start declining until thirty or forty seconds after the activity that triggered the decline begins.

It takes the body an appreciable amount of time to accommodate a new set of conditions. For example, one cannot sit in a car for any period of time, exit the car, and start walking and expect the blood oxygen content to remain stable. It will drop until the heart and lungs adapt to the new set of conditions, in this case, walking.

Breathing in through the nose and exhaling through the mouth, as opposed to both inhaling and exhaling through the nose, is very desirable; it can increase blood oxygen saturation by as much as two percent. In the past fifteen months, I have learned a lot, and I am still learning.

Most importantly, I have learned to fight pulmonary fibrosis without giving up all the activities I once enjoyed. My pulmonary performance is better now than it was in July 2000. I do not think I will be dying soon!

I plan to go snowboarding this winter and to go camping and fishing in Baja next spring. Life still stretches out before me. I think that you can also make similar strides, if you are determined to do so. Do not give up!

◆ ❖ ◆

Sue Ann Kulcsar
Son with Scleredema
Ohio, USA

Scleredema is an illness similar to scleroderma. It is also known as Scleredema Adultorum, Scleredema Adultorum of Buschke, Scleredema Diabeticorum, and Scleredema Diabeticorum of Buschke. This is a very rare disease. Up to 1965, only two hundred twenty-three cases of scleredema had been reported worldwide.

My son went off to college in the fall of 1998. When he returned a month later, his face had started to thicken by the bridge of his nose. Soon his face was thick by his cheeks and eyes. He went from doctor to doctor. In December 1999, he was hospitalized with a heart problem: multifocal atrial tachycardia.

He kept going to different doctors. An X ray and CT scan showed his lungs were beginning to thicken. In September 2000, he was hospitalized three times for this heart problem. He would wake up in the morning and his resting heart rate would be about one hundred thirty beats per minute. He is now on a heart medication that makes him agitated at times.

His face continues to thicken. He has had two biopsies that came back confirming scleredema. This is hard on all of us because his older sister had a rare brain tumor in 1981. She has many problems caused by radiation damage. My son's doctors want to try chemotherapy and then irradiate his face. But after seeing the problems my daughter has had from radiation, I do not want to subject my son to that.

Since Christmas of 2000, the left side of my son's face thickened even more. On February 9, he was told he has cataracts in both eyes. He had just had an eye exam in December, and his eyes were fine.

The cardiologist said the next time that my son's heart beats irregularly for more than several hours, they will open up his heart to find out what is wrong with it.

◆ ❖ ◆

Franco Pilone
Italy

I am fifty-seven years old, and three years ago I was diagnosed with Sjögren's syndrome but, in reality, I have been suffering from it for almost thirty years. Before the final diagnosis, my doctor sent me for numerous specific tests, after which he drew his conclusions.

Ten years ago, I had autoimmune pericarditis. I suffered so much! I took various medicines, but the problem did not clear up. Three years ago, I underwent a pericardectomy and I hoped that everything would be resolved; instead I continue to have chest pain and I still can't cope without taking steroids for it.

I have had salivary gland biopsies. I am suffering from rheumatoid arthritis, and I have serious problems with my eyes. The lack of tears has caused inflammation of the corneas. I have strong pain and intestinal problems, all due to Sjögren's Syndrome. I often get tired when I walk a bit quickly or after any effort.

Currently, I am under the care of an immunologist at Niguarda Hospital in Milan, and I am taking many medications including painkillers when needed. Despite all these problems, I nonetheless go forward with the hope that a treatment for this disease will be found.

◆ ❖ ◆

V. O.
Italy

I am a thirty-year-old woman, and I have been suffering for three years from Sjögren's syndrome with highly positive anti-SSA antibodies.

I am being treated with cortisone, and about a year ago a monoclonal immunoglobulin peak appeared in my blood. I continue to take the same cortisone treatment although recently, after a stressful episode, my symptoms worsened, with pain in my right parotid gland. This resolved after the dose of steroid was increased.

I am very worried about my condition. I am a member of our local association, but this has not been a great help. I would like to get in contact with other colleagues (in fact, I am a doctor) who could help me and, above all, share with me their experiences.

I would also like to have information about the possibility of getting pregnant, and about the likelihood of developing a malignancy.

Maureen Thomason
Daughter Alexa, Undiagnosed
California, USA

We have an eight-year-old daughter whose symptoms have stumped our pediatrician. On two fingers of her right hand, she has redness and bumps that do not itch and are not painful.

She is nauseated on and off all day. She has a pimple-like bump in the corner of her mouth and a new white bump on the tip of her tongue. She says she is hungry all the time but cannot eat. Her tummy feels heavy. She gets pains now and then in her lower right side or in different places, and she has heartburn.

About six months ago, she would be playing and suddenly have to sit down, complaining that her heart was beating too fast and that she did not feel well. This went on for weeks. She had an EKG and an echocardiogram that both showed nothing.

The finger rash, oddly, appears and disappears. The first time, it turned wrinkly and then faded away when she was put on antibiotics for pharyngitis. On that visit with another doctor, we were told the rash was eczema. Later, the same rash appeared again, only this time the left index finger had a swelling on the right side that made her finger look crooked. It too went away. Again, the rash came back on the same two fingers. No swelling this time, just red with pimple-like bumps and no itching or pain. She was increasingly nauseated throughout the day.

Her blood test was positive for ANA. All else was well. She had her hands X rayed. Nothing was there. She was taken off milk products for a week. No real improvement. She is now on a gluten-free diet. Maybe it is too soon to tell.

We do not know what is going on with her. The doctor will be sending her to a gastroenterologist in a couple of weeks. At the time she saw the rheumatologist, the rash was gone, so he did not have much to say.

I know the rash is not the typical scleroderma rash, and she does not have symptoms of Raynaud's phenomenon; however, the traveling pain, the nausea, and the heart and stomach problems make me wonder if these are the symptoms of systemic scleroderma. I read that early symptoms of progressive systemic scleroderma in juveniles differ from adults; however,

I cannot find specific descriptions of those symptoms. Our doctor is now checking for celiac disease.

Do any of these symptoms ring a bell? I am looking for a lead to follow.

Update – August 2001

We still do not know what's up. We were referred to a dermatologist. He said that it looked like lupus and ordered an extensive blood panel. We were then sent to a rheumatologist, who was very thorough in his explanation as to why he felt Alexa did not have an autoimmune disease. He said that her ANA was very low, and all the other tests were negative. He believes the heartburn and nausea problems are unrelated to the rash on her fingers. He said the pains in her joints and the cracking of her knuckles were normal. He tested her flexibility and said it was excellent.

So the next stop was the gastroenterologist. Weeks and sometimes months would pass before we could see these doctors. It was a tough waiting game. Prior to the gastroenterologist's appointment, Alexa was put on medication which helped with the heartburn a bit. The nausea did not occur as often. To this day, the rash appears and disappears. The gastroenterologist did a barium test and an ultrasound—both clear. The endoscopy showed red irritation at the duodenum. We waited another week to see if she had a parasite. That was negative; the esophagus was fine.

The gastroenterologist put Alexa on another medication in hope that within a month, whatever was causing the irritation would clear up.

The rash reappeared and because of our health insurance, we had to go back to the same dermatologist for a second opinion before we could go to the specific dermatologist to whom the rheumatologist referred us. This time, the dermatologist (same office, but different doctor) scheduled another battery of blood tests and said that he wanted to be sure it was not scleroderma.

Ironically, I had pushed the first dermatologist to test for scleroderma, but he said that it was extremely rare. He quickly flashed me a picture of a patient with an advanced case on her hands and said that it was more like lupus. He left in a hurry. When I looked over the blood tests he was ordering, I noticed the word "CREST."

After the rheumatologist's opinion and the gastroenterologist's opinion, this dermatologist, who did not have a copy of prior blood work, wanted to test for scleroderma. We had to wait another week because we wanted the pediatrician to check over the tests to be sure they had not already been administered. The pediatrician went on vacation for two weeks; the gastroenterologist went for three.

Now we have an appointment with the gastroenterologist to let him know the medication has not solved the problem completely. Although Alexa has nausea less frequently, she has pain in her chest at times, and still has heartburn. That rash has now disappeared. The "eat-a-radioactive-sandwich test" may be next. It will be another two weeks before we can talk to the gastroenterologist at Loma Linda Hospital. He is very professional, but very busy!

The blessing in all of this is that Alexa experiences illness in bouts, and then it goes away. For the most part, Alexa is highly energetic, strong, and happy. She even beat her twelve-year-old brother in a push-up competition!

Update – February 2002

Alexa passed the "sandwich test" with flying colors. The gastroenterologist said the tests beyond this one are painful, so he is going to wait. He gave her another prescription and another appointment in two months, which was delayed because the doctor was on vacation again.

The same symptoms come and go and overlap. Hardly a day goes by without nausea or heartburn. She complains of pain in the area of her duodenum and around the area of her heart (so she describes). These pains come and go. Sometimes, with no activity, her heartbeat starts racing. When the rash appears on her fingers, it constantly changes. It does not look the same at night as it did that morning.

I called the gastroenterologist to let him know that Alexa felt no difference in spite of the prescriptions, and that I was seeing a definite link between the presence of the rash and the intensity of the other symptoms. He said to take her to the dermatologist the next time the rash broke out, have a biopsy done, and send him the results. He gave us another prescription. He had always believed that Alexa's gastrointestinal symptoms were separate from the rash symptoms; he now believed she may have some type of autoimmune disease.

It is heartbreaking to watch your child suffer and not be able to do anything to relieve it. It is so frustrating to deal with the HMO system. We were just informed that in order to see the dermatologist we prefer, it requires that our current dermatologist write a letter stating there is nothing more he can do. The HMO says that that never happens.

Last week was really tough. Alexa's symptoms have intensified. In spite of her extreme nausea, she pushes herself to get through her school days. She will have bouts that come and go. On February 13, she tripped while walking up the stairs at school to her classroom. We spent five hours in urgent care to get an X ray of her ankle. To make a long story short, Alexa now has a cast on her left leg and yet another doctor is added to the chain; a podiatrist.

Our little girl is truly a trooper. She does not let her battle with this mysterious illness knock her down. In spite of the daily visits to the nurse's office, she has managed to be an honor roll student. Alexa is an inspiration, and we know that there is a purpose in all of this.

Update

Alexa's illness has completely resolved itself, having disappeared about as suddenly as it had started. We are and thankful for our faith, which gave us peace and sustained us through her illness.

CHAPTER 8

Overlap, UCTD and MCTD Stories

I found I am not alone.
— Kellie Kennedy

Cindy
Undifferentiated Connective Tissue Disease (UCTD)
Texas, USA

I am thirty-six years old. I was diagnosed, if you can call it that, with undifferentiated connective tissue disease (UCTD) when I was thirty. I was ten, though, when things started happening. I was told I had juvenile rheumatoid arthritis (JRA). The doctors advised my mom to treat it with aspirin and exercise.

When I was thirty and working in an emergency room, I began to get sick often. I was hurting and aching a lot. I just wanted to lie down and sleep as soon as I got home from work, which was difficult with two very small children.

Since then, I have had to stop working. I may have a few good days where I am able to do a lot, and then I will have even more bad days making up for it. Holding down a steady job has not been possible. I am in my second year of trying to be approved for Social Security Disability. I would much rather be able to work as I miss it a lot, but I know that it will completely wear me down.

On those days when I feel good, thoughts of, "I should be working like everyone else," can take over and then a few days later, I am back to, "What was I thinking?" Does this sound familiar? Wouldn't it be nice if those of us with this disease could job-share? When you are feeling good, you work, and then I will take over the next week and so on. Perhaps this is just a wish to be back in the real world.

Following my divorce, I went for over a year with no medication and no financial resources to see a rheumatologist. I had lost my health insurance with the divorce. It took me more than a year to get into an indigent-care program (what a horrible-sounding term). Now I am on several medications, which seem to be working somewhat.

The symptoms I have now are pain and stiffness in my feet, ankles, hips, hands, and wrists. My shoulders are beginning to bother me as well. I have visual disturbances where I see sparkles. I have tension headaches and a horrible rash on my arms and torso if I am exposed to the sun without sun block.

I also have little red dots (petechiae) on my skin, and I get rashes and little bumps, almost like knots, under my skin. I always run a low-grade fever. For the past couple of weeks, I have been extremely tired again, wanting to sleep a lot, and I have an extremely difficult time waking up in the morning.

The rheumatologist I see now seems to think I have systemic lupus erythematosus (SLE). I have negative rheumatoid factor with positive anti-nuclear antibodies (ANA), but until my symptoms better match the criteria for SLE, he cannot make a definitive diagnosis.

He says treatment for undifferentiated connective tissue disease (UCTD) and SLE is the same, so it does not matter what it is called. I agree. So that is my story.

Kellie Kennedy
Thyroid Cancer, Sjögren's, Raynaud's, Underlying Scleroderma
California, USA

I recently came across www.sclero.org when I began researching my longterm illness. I was so relieved to read about many people who have had the same experiences and symptoms as me. Not that I wished this on anyone, but I was not alone!

In 1993, I developed toxic shock syndrome (TSS). At the time, I thought it was a bad case of the flu. By the third day, a friend came over to bring cold medicine only to see how sick I looked. He told me he was taking me to the emergency room. I was lucky, because I was near death, and he saved my life.

After going through TSS, I never felt good from that moment on. I always caught anything and everything you could catch. My body began to change and slow down.

By 1996, I really was not feeling well. I went to my gynecologist as my periods were very irregular, and they had always been like a clock. The doctor claimed my thyroid was out of control and he could not understand how I was even walking around.

Although he never did a complete examination, the doctor prescribed thyroid medication. After a few months on it, I felt no different. I returned to the doctor weekly, complaining of weight loss, seizures, and extreme sensitivity to cold. The doctor ignored those symptoms.

One day, I noticed my neck was swollen and when I swallowed, I noticed a lump. Through my insurance plan, I requested a different endocrinologist, who immediately scheduled the correct procedures to find out whether the lump was a tumor. The initial findings were that it was.

The next step was to rule out cancer. After much consultation, I decided to have a needle biopsy before agreeing to surgery. I had been warned that needle biopsies are often not conclusive, which was the case with my biopsy. But the doctors agreed the tumor had to come out. I was scheduled for surgery to remove half my thyroid. The doctor told me the odds of the tumor being cancer were pretty low.

Five days after surgery, the doctor informed me it was papillary/ follicular cancer, a rare combination of aggressive and nonaggressive cancer. The next day I had surgery to remove the remaining half of my thyroid. During that time, I was also diagnosed with the autoimmune disease,

Hashimoto's thyroiditis. It is rare to have an autoimmune disease and cancer at the same time. I was told nothing much could be done about the Hashimoto's except live with it. Does that sound familiar to any of you?

I was also diagnosed with fibromyalgia. So I was completely devastated by all the news. All that time I was never referred to any type of support group. After my thyroidectomy, I was never given any postsurgical advice on how to cope without my thyroid. For women, it is critical to regulating metabolism and other bodily functions. Doctors only told me, "You should start to feel better once your body gets regulated to the medication."

Needless to say, three years later, I feel just as bad as I did before the cancer, and my medication never seems to regulate anything. I should mention that during this entire ordeal I was fighting with my health plan on what they would approve, which was very stressful and did nothing to help me mentally.

After flip-flopping from one endocrinologist to another, I ended up with one I liked. She always listened to what I told her about my thyroid, but she was not aggressive in finding out why my arms and legs were numb and burning. No part of my body was pain free. I also told her my energy level was at an all-time low. I used to be very active in all sports and now just walking a flight of stairs was almost impossible.

By strange luck, my insurance changed again and I was not able to continue seeing her. I ended up at another clinic here in Los Angeles. I do like my doctors but still, they never go that extra mile to investigate my symptoms.

I recently started having digestive and severe swallowing problems. I underwent a very uncomfortable procedure with the camera down the nose and throat. I have a seven-second-plus delay in swallowing (most people swallow in under two seconds). The doctors had no explanation other than they think a main muscle may have been disturbed during the thyroidectomy.

I have major dental problems. My teeth break at a drop of a dime, and I have TMJ to top it off. I have positive antinuclear antibodies (ANA) for lupus and Sjögren's syndrome fifty percent of the time—and they cannot tell me what is going on.

My personality has completely changed. My anger has come out in very negative ways. I knew it but did not know what to do about it. People were telling me things about my personality that just did not reflect who I was all these years.

This devastated me. A man who had become very special to me, recently told me that the anger I directed toward him and my overbearing personality were just not working for him. I sat there and cried. Was he really talking about me? My anger was how I coped with my illness, yet I did not know how or whom to talk to about it. I was mad at him for not being able to spot it, to recognize it. How could he?

Growing up, I was always the one with no temper and was anything but overbearing. Needless to say, our relationship became an often-strained friendship. Understandably, my anger made it almost impossible for him to get close to me. It makes me very sad, more than he will ever know.

My illness played a major role in that relationship's demise because I waited too long to seek help for my anger. I did enter therapy to address the anger issues, and that was when I started to research scleroderma.

Information from the www.sclero.org website led me to Dr. Daniel Wallace, a scleroderma specialist here in Los Angeles, to find out if I do indeed have scleroderma and, if not, what exactly my body was doing. I will also be joining an autoimmune support group.

An autoimmune disease is very debilitating and plays havoc with your mental state. Nobody should have to go through what I have without some type of support group. People with illnesses, such as cancer and autoimmune disease, often stop talking to their friends and family members for fear nobody understands or wants to hear about it anymore, which is devastating.

Update – May 2000

I have been diagnosed with Raynaud's phenomenon and Sjögren's and am in the long process of trying to determine if I have scleroderma. In the last month, I have had a pulmonary function test (PFT), CT scan, and an echocardiogram. None of these tests are showing the doctors the conclusive evidence they need to diagnose scleroderma.

I am scheduled for a pulmonary exercise test next week to see why I am having such difficult time breathing. I have extreme pains in the left side of my chest. I am barely able to walk up a flight of stairs without being winded and tired, and my arms and legs feel like lead.

I was put on medication for the Raynaud's phenomenon, but was taken off it after two days because my blood pressure dropped too low. Now I'm on an arthritis pain medication to help with the inflammation. So far, I've been able to tolerate it. I am very frustrated and stressed, as you can imagine.

Update – September 2000

It can be so overwhelming: thyroidectomy, Sjögren's, Raynaud's phenomenon, early signs of scleroderma, Hashimoto's thyroiditis, and fibromyalgia.

I just had a complete MRI done on my brain and spine. They thought I might have lesions because of the numbness I have all the time and the lack of use of my left side most of the time. My symptoms include fatigue; blurred vision; numbness in arms, legs, and fingers; severe joint pain where I can hardly walk or lay down; shortness of breath, and headaches.

Although I try to stay off medication as much as I can, I take medicines for my thyroid, Sjögren's, and migraine headaches. My mood swings were really bad prior to medication. I did join a support group in Los Angeles and got online with people. I am still in therapy to talk about my feelings.

My neurologist found that due to Sjögren's, the gel-like substance between my vertebrae is being destroyed. I am beginning physical therapy, which will help slow this down. Exercise is a catch twenty-two: if I feel good enough to do it, I am in severe pain afterward. That is why I will start physical therapy so I can start to rebuild my body.

I am very lucky as I still work and have a crazy schedule. I raise money for a major children's hospital here in Los Angeles. I have to be in front of people every day putting on a happy smile.

Update – January 2002

After two more years of getting sicker and weaker with increased headaches, complete loss of movement of my left arm, partial loss of movement to the left leg as well as memory loss, I finally took matters into my own hands. I went to see one of the top scleroderma specialists at University of California, Los Angeles (UCLA), regardless of what my insurance plan approved. This specialist believed I may have lupus along with the Sjögren's and Raynaud's phenomenon. He advised me that I might have what is called secondary or underlying scleroderma, often associated with Sjögren's, but not full-blown.

He sent me to a top lupus doctor, and I was diagnosed with borderline symptoms of lupus. The lupus specialist was not convinced of full-blown lupus. He advised that he would watch me carefully and referred me to a top doctor at Scripps Clinic in San Diego who handled Sjögren's to see if the headaches and loss of movement on my left side and loss of memory were related to Sjögren's.

While at Scripps Clinic, I was diagnosed with seizures and small strokes, also known as transient ischemic attacks (TIAs). In the opinion of the doctor at Scripps, a thirty-nine-year-old woman should not have near complete loss of control of her left side and memory loss, and this was not being caused by the Sjögren's, but by something else.

They sent me back to a top neurologist where I had an MRI, spinal taps, and PET scans. I was diagnosed with one band of multiple sclerosis (MS), although the doctors felt that could be disregarded as many patients with autoimmune disease have at least one band of MS show in a spinal tap. They also discovered a problem with the frontal lobe of my brain, as seen in patients with autoimmune and other serious diseases.

After many more tests, it was determined the TIAs were due to an overproduction of calcium, which does not allow the blood to flow freely. I was prescribed a calcium channel blocker and one baby aspirin a day with my other medications. I was placed into two months of physical therapy to regain the use of my left side. As a result, I was out of work for two and a half months.

After finding out how I had been misdiagnosed by the doctors in my health plan, I wrote a letter of appeal to my insurance company demanding they reverse the ruling and pick up all costs. I received an apology letter and the reverse ruling from them.

You have to fight for everything with the insurance company or you will get nothing approved! Trust me! I have fought for everything and had to follow up on referrals, and so on.

It is helpful to have our friends and family read as much as possible about our illnesses. It helps them understand the disease and what we are feeling, and it provides them tips on dealing with it.

I have my good days and my bad days. Soon I will be forty years old and my doctors say they have never seen a patient with all these diseases look so good. I still exercise. I eat well with a low-carbohydrate diet, and I still work full time.

I would like to thank my friend, Natasha, for suggesting I submit this story. Working is a double-edged sword. I work for the City of Hope Cancer Medical Center in Los Angeles. I am lucky, because they have been supportive and understanding. We have a saying at City of Hope, "There is always hope." I truly believe that!

◆ ❖ ◆

Krista Lurtz
Scleroderma, Polymyositis, Vasculitis
Romania

When this was written, Krista lived in Qatar, far away from her family and friends. Now she is back home in Romania. Krista's story is also in Romanian, later in this book.

I promised Shelley Ensz that some day I would try to write my real story. It has been some time since that day. I tried, yes, I did, but something kept me from doing it.

Many of you may know that I have translated web pages on the www. sclero.org website into my language of Romanian. Before the accuracy of my medical translations was confirmed by medical professionals in my country, I felt my translations were poor for two reasons:

1. I did not have any Romanian documents to help me. I spent a lot of time working on the translations. After two years of speaking English, it was not easy to start translating words that I had never heard in my own language, especially when I had no dictionary. However, I did not give up. I know it is not a perfect translation, but at least it is something! Shelley knows that prior to my translated pages, if someone tried to find something about scleroderma or any of these problems in Romanian on the Internet, it was impossible because there was nothing there. When I started, I was hungry for knowledge, yet I was depressed, upset, and lonely, far from home, far from family. It was hard for me to look for all the information and find it in a foreign language.

2. There is not much to say! I know everyone wishes there was something to give hope! However, there is nothing. The hope is not in the medical books; the hope is in us! Medically, you can say everything about it in just few words: "We do not know where the disease comes from. We do not know the treatment." That is all. The rest is how lucky we are to have a good doctor, to get the diagnosis, and to have the symptoms treated.

Me? I have no doctor! I have my pills in the house, and I am afraid to use them because I do not have any idea how to control them! Mostly, I am very scared about the side effects. And I do not have anyone beside me to give me real support. I hope that I have enough energy to make it like this until the summer when I am going home to my doctors, and we will start a treatment.

The story? I am reading all the other stories and for every one I am thinking, "What is behind these words?" How much pain? How many minutes of loneliness? How many hurts are inside that person who feels it is so hard to go on? How much does it hurt that we cannot walk or sleep, or eat? How much energy can we put into covering our pains with a smile?

How much does it hurt inside? Not the physical pain. That pain is there. Take a pill, and it may make you feel better. But how many tears are we crying in the night? I cannot stop myself thinking about that.

We are doing the best that we can. We are writing stories, personal stories, using the words that do not hurt the one who is reading it too much. We are careful to not complain too much.

We are just trying our best to help in some way with simple words, which mean so much. We just do not say it all. We do not say how much it hurts. We do not say anything about that scream inside of us. On the other hand, it is not right to have nights when we are filled with fear.

In addition to translating, I have written many personal pages in Romanian for the website. I do my best to put in a lot of feelings. I have some humor there, too. Moreover, some articles contain the way life is, or is not.

The big surprise I have had from my personal pages is the emails from people who are healthy, and they tell me that my pages help them to better understand the meaning of life. These are people who do not really know the pain, but they feel that life is not fair to them. They tell me that my words help them to understand that they are selfish and not thinking, that life can be really unfair to someone else.

I am happy. I am really happy. I do help people!

Today, I will start another chapter in my page. In addition, I will be writing about all the pain: the fears and the tears inside of me. It is hard to open up. The ones around us will never know how to become closer to us. They want to. They do want to understand why we are crying when there is nothing to cry about. They need help to understand why we are angry for no reason or why yesterday we laughed, but today we are so sad. Why we get upset when they say we are looking well.

I want to let them know why sometimes I do not feel like having anyone around. Those are the moments when my spirit screams at life. I have no energy to smile or to take life as it is. I must do it, I will do it, but I do have moments when I prefer to see this earth crumble into small pieces.

They all are looking at me like I am such a brave person. I want to let them know that I am not! I am as simple as they are. Life put me in a position I never asked for. I am not a hero. I am simply the product of my pain.

That is all I am. Moreover, I am doing my best to help everyone, no matter if they are healthy or not. We all need help. And the help is inside us. We just have to learn how to let it come out. That is all. Is it too much? Not enough? I will never know. I only hope that my words will help some more people.

Mick
Undifferentiated Connective Tissue Disease, Lupus
South Dakota, USA

Regardless of what gender my name falls under, I am a female who has struggled for the past five to six years to get a straight diagnosis. I have been to countless doctors with my many symptoms, which include joint and muscle aches and pains, fatigue, rashes, swelling, and many others. At first, I thought I was losing my mind.

I started with my family doctor and from there, I became very frustrated and very untrusting of medical personnel. First I came across one nasty nurse, then a bookkeeper that could not get my account straightened out, followed by doctors who continually asked if I drank too much and how much did I smoke, and who told me, "We think you are depressed!" I felt I was being treated as some dumb blonde.

Finally, one day I was referred to a rheumatologist. That was five or six years ago, and I am still being told different things: one time I have lupus, and the next time I have undifferentiated connective tissue disease (UCTD). All this simply means is they are not entirely sure yet which CTD it is.

Some of the doctors have said to me, "Oh, you do not want to have lupus or scleroderma." Duh! Now is there some reason I would want one of these diseases? I just want to know what is wrong, and what to expect!

So I know how it feels to feel like an outcast, but dealing with this disease is not nearly as bad as dealing with the question: "What is this disease?"

I have created a site on the Internet for people like me: Mick's UCTD and Autoimmune Site. I have researched and found links on many autoimmune diseases. You can search on symptoms to gain knowledge and understanding of autoimmune diseases. Then you can take the information to your next doctor appointment and have an informed discussion with your doctor. My site is for informational purposes only, and is not a substitute for appropriate medical care.

◆ ❖ ◆

Nan
Mixed Connective Tissue Disease, Fibromyalgia
Ohio, USA

I have always been an active person, raising four children alone after a fifteen-year marriage dissolved. I prided myself on being listed as the seventh woman in the state of Ohio to become a cement finisher apprentice with the Local 886 out of Toledo, Ohio. With a love of horses since childhood, I gave riding lessons in Western, English, and Huntseat.

During these early years, I began to draw again and designed a line of greeting cards called *Use Caution Concepts*. I resigned from the cement-finishing program when my health and children's issues began to creep in. We moved to a smaller community south of Toledo in early 1992.

Not long after having my fourth child, I began to experience symptoms similar to those of multiple sclerosis (MS). I spent many years in and out of different medical centers trying to find out the cause. I was told many times to talk with a psychiatrist. I always agreed, yet the psychiatrists kept sending me back to the medical doctors. I had developed different types of skin growths that the local pathology group could not diagnose after a week of study.

I had been raised with a father who was a radiologist. Thank goodness for his keen insight and wisdom. He knew there was something going on, so he never let me give up. Raised around medical professionals, I had a different approach to doctors than most. I became aggressive after about the fifth diagnosis of fibromyalgia and demanded medical treatment.

One other odd thing with this mixed connective tissue disease (MCTD) is that I had a strange growth removed by my primary doctor at Ohio State University (OSU). It showed positive for only connective tissue! I have had blood tests often come back showing high titers, an electroprotein immunoglobulinemia spike, and a mild-to-moderate-range Epstein-Barr.

Finally, after several years of struggle, one wonderful doctor at OSU got gutsy and gave me the MCTD diagnosis. This past summer I had some female surgery, and the chart read, "Blunt force and sharp force needed to remove." My gynecologist said, "It was the MCTD that made removal difficult."

There are new diagnoses now on my basic medical forms. I have applied for disability in Ohio and have been denied several times. I cannot work; the drug labels alone advise that one should not drive.

I am very limited in what I can do. One day may be good but then the next three are bad. I need my gallbladder out, but I have postponed that because my blood pressure has to get stabilized first. I just underwent a cardio stress test and am relieved to know my heart is okay at this time.

I want to thank you for letting me share part of my story. I have some suggestions for those who are not only saddled with chronic illness, but may also have problems finding proper caregivers.

1. Be aggressive.

2. Find at least two primary doctors who will work together for you.

3. Build a team of doctors who will understand the complexity of your illness.

4. Keep a list of all necessary telephone numbers well within reach and on your person. I also suggest giving the list to each doctor.

5. Build a file. Each time there is a new or different test, get the results, and give copies to each doctor, and keep a copy for yourself, too!

6. Each doctor needs your prescription list.

7. Get all your prescriptions from the same pharmacy.

8. Build a relationship with at least one of the people who fill your prescriptions.

9. Make sure you wear a medical bracelet if your doctors feel it necessary.

10. File for disability if your doctor says you are disabled. Do it fast! The process of applying and review can take years. Who knows where you will be by then.

11. Continue to love and enjoy your family and friends. They are going through this with you.

Bright blessings to you all!

◆ ❖ ◆

Shar
Lupus, Scleroderma, Sjögren's, Fibromyalgia
Arizona, USA

One day in October of 1998, at 11:00 P.M., I was on the phone with my sister-in-law when I suddenly got a sharp pain in my upper abdomen. Within fifteen minutes, I was really feeling ill. Two days later, after tubes and tubes of blood, MRIs and body scans, the doctor delivered the news that I was hepatitis C (HCV) positive, my gallbladder had been destroyed and needed to be removed, my liver was one step from cirrhosis, and my terrible body pain was caused by fibromyalgia. I had gone from being well to being very ill in the blink of an eye.

Only a few months earlier, I had had my annual physical exam, and all was clear. I was one of those with HCV who never had an abnormal liver test. I have no history of drinking or drugs, but I am a nurse with a history of accidental needle sticks and blood spills, and now I am the patient.

Due to the condition of my liver, I underwent forty-seven weeks of daily hepatitis treatments. It was a horrid experience! I suffered brain fog, hair loss, body pain, extreme weight loss, and fatigue. Both the HCV and the medications opened the floodgate for autoimmune disease with a fury. Within six weeks, I was in full HCV remission, but I had to continue therapy to make sure it did not return. My choices were few: cirrhosis or autoimmune disease.

My first autoimmune symptoms included the terrible facial butterfly rash of lupus. This appeared along with the nodules of rheumatoid arthritis (RA) on my legs, accompanied by neuropathy in my feet and protein in my urine. The list of symptoms and lab findings seems to be endless: short-term memory loss; facial, forearm, hands, and lower extremity skin thickening; and some facial bone loss. Sjögren's has caused many problems with my teeth. Constant irritable bowel syndrome (IBS) often keeps me homebound. The butterfly rash has settled into a permanent blush.

Two months ago, I underwent successful lithotripsy for a large kidney stone. My urine is still protein positive, and I await the results of a twenty-four-hour urine test, while they check for the cause of the stone and the condition of my kidneys.

My white blood count is inexplicably high. I have a lovely new cough, and I am now on medications for heart palpitations, a dynamic heartbeat, and hypertension. My primary care physician and rheumatologist have prescribed medicines to control the outrageous neuropathy, fibromyalgia, and rheumatoid arthritis, as well as the scleroderma muscle and joint pain. I still lose hair and have unreal scalp sensitivity. It seems like I have yet to not be in a flare, and sleep is evasive at best, but the HCV remains in remission.

Was my battle with HCV worth it? Yes! I forgive myself for those days I refer to as my daze. Now I set one goal to accomplish each day, even if it is just doing a load of laundry. I have two great kids—the best reasons to fight on.

PART 4

International

CHAPTER 9

Greek

Dimitra Stafilia
United Kingdom (Greece)

Dimitra Stafilia is ISN's Greek Translator. The English translation of this story is in Chapter 2.

Η μητέρα μου διαγνώστηκε με σκληρόδερμα για πρώτη φορά το 1992. Όλα άρχισαν με έναν οξύ πόνο στα δάχτυλά της. Όταν άρχιζε να κάνει κρύο ή όταν έβαζε τα χέρια της κάτω από κρύο νερό, τα δάχτυλά της μελάνιαζαν και μετά άσπριζαν. Αποφάσισε να πάει σε αγγειολόγο ο οποίος διαπίστωσε στένωση των αιμοφόρων αγγείων. Ο αγγειολόγος της, θέλοντας να εξετάσει όλες τις περιπτώσεις, την παρέπεμψε σε ένα ρευματολόγο ο οποίος και διέγνωσε την ασθένειά της. Τουλάχιστον η μητέρα μου ήταν τυχερή και οι γιατροί της εξέτασαν όλες τις εκδοχές.

Η ασθένεια της μητέρας μου άλλαξε την ζωή για όλη την οικογένεια. Κανείς μας δεν ήξερε τι ήταν, πως προκλήθηκε ή πόσο σοβαρό ήταν. Πώς λέμε «ο αόρατος εχθρός»; Εγώ ήμουν ακόμα στο λύκειο και ούτε που μπορούσα να καταλάβω πόσο επώδυνο θα ήταν. Το πρώτο πράγμα που έκανε η μητέρα μου ήταν να αρχίσει να διαβάζει και να μαθαίνει για την αρρώστια της. Το 1992 η χρήση του Internet στην Ελλάδα δεν ήταν τόσο διαδεδομένη και οι μόνες πηγές πληροφόρησης ήταν οι εγκυκλοπαίδειες και η θεία μου στη Νέα Υόρκη.

Από που ήρθε αυτή η αρρώστα; Έχω διαβάσει άρθρα που λένε ότι μπορεί να οφείλεται σε περιβαλλοντικούς ή γενετικούς παράγοντες. Η οικογένεια μου έζησε για πολλά χρόνια εντός μιας βιομηχανικής ζώνης. Ο πατέρας μου, μέχρι την συνταξιοδότησή του πριν από 4 χρόνια, δούλευε για μια εταιρεία παραγωγής σιδηρονικελίου. (Το χώμα από τα ορυχεία περιείχε επίσης μικρές ποσότητες κοβαλτίου και χαλκού, τις οποίες διεχώριζαν και μετά πετούσαν σαν σκουριά). Δεν ξέρω κανέναν άλλο από την περιοχή αυτή που να έχει σκληρόδερμα, αλλά πάλι εμείς μείναμε μερικά χρόνια παραπάνω από την πλειονότητα των εργαζομένων εκεί.

Με τα χρόνια η νόσος προχωρούσε άσχημα. Τα δάχτυλά της ήταν πρησμένα στις αρθρώσεις και δεν μπορούσε να τα λυγίσει, τα νύχια της σχίζονταν και μπορούσες να δεις την σάρκα από κάτω τους. Είχε πνευμονική ίνωση, προβλήματα με τον οισοφάγο, υπέρταση και δύσπνοια. Και αυτά είναι μόνο μερικά από τα προβλήματά της. Για να καταπολεμήσει τα ανεξάρτητα συμπτώματα παίρνει ένα κοκτέιλ φαρμάκων και επισκέπτεται τακτικά εξειδικευμένους γιατρούς (ανάλογα με το πρόβλημα) για να ελέγξει την καρδιά και τους πνεύμονές της, ενώ έχει ένα γιατρό που επιβλέπει την όλη αγωγή της. Η χρήση της κορτιζόνης για την πνευμονική ίνωση της προκάλεσε οστεοπόρωση (ακόμα στα αρχικά στάδια). Επίσης, εξαιτίας της, είναι υπέρβαρη, κάτι που χειροτερεύει την κατάστασή της. Η μητέρα μου είναι 51 ετών. Προσωπικά άρχισα να ερευνώ τη νόσο όταν πήγα πανεπιστήμιο. Όταν αργότερα ήρθα στην Αγγλία επισκέφθηκα το νοσοκομείο Royal Free Hospital στο Λονδίνο, και έγραψα στην Αμερικανική Ένωση Σκληροδέρματος (American Scleroderma Association) για ένα ενημερωτικό πακέτο. Ωστόσο δεν υπήρχε τίποτα στα ελληνικά. Ούτε άρθρα, ούτε ομάδες υποστήριξης των ασθενών και δεν υπήρχε τρόπος να ξέρω αν ο γιατρός της γνώριζε τις τελευταίες ιατρικές εξελίξεις ή αν της ζητούσε να κάνει τα σωστά τεστ. Πιστεύω ότι οι ασθενείς πρέπει να γνωρίζουν την κατάστασή τους ώστε να μπορούν να ελέγχουν αλλά και να βοηθούν τον γιατρό τους. Αυτό δεν συνέβη με την μητέρα μου. Για αυτό λοιπόν ενδιαφέρομαι να μεταφράσω τις σελίδες του Scleroderma from A to Z. Θέλω να δώσω και στους άλλους Έλληνες ασθενείς τη δυνατότητα να μάθουν κάτι παραπάνω αλλά και να ξέρουν ότι υπάρχουν και άλλοι με τα ίδια προβλήματα.

Όσο για εμένα, είμαι μεταφράστρια και εργάζομαι στο Λονδίνο ως project manager. Ακόμα πιστεύω ότι παρά τις ακαδημαϊκές ή επαγγελματικές επιτυχίες μου, δεν έχω κάνει αρκετά για την μητέρα μου, και αφού βρίσκομαι μακριά της και δεν μπορώ να την στηρίξω, αυτή είναι η μικρή συνεισφορά μου.

CHAPTER 10

Italiano (Italian)

Angiola Sbolli
Italy

The English version of this story is in Chapter 3.

La sclerosi sistemica progressiva è stata riscontrata nel febbraio 1997, all'età di cinquantasette anni. La diagnosi è stata immediata, al momento della prima visita, in quanto i segni della malattia, in stato già avanzato, erano molto evidenti.

Già da molti anni erano presenti i sintomi che ho trascurato per lungo tempo: l'ispessimento della cute dell'addome; il gonfiore e il dolore delle mani, con rigidità ed ulcerazioni; una tosse persistente e generale spossamento fisico. Dopo una fase acuta, oggi (aprile 2000) sembra che la malattia si sia, per il momento, stabilizzata, ma i danni non si sono risolti: soffro di una fibrosi polmonare di marcata entità che mi costringe all'uso continuo di ossigeno, un'esofagite da reflusso, un lieve coinvolgimento cardiaco ed una grave compromissione viscerale e dolori diffusi.

Assumo terapia con steroidi e nifedipina che ha decisamente migliorato lo stato delle mie mani colpite dal fenomeno di Raynaud.

Questa è la mia storia, mi piacerebbe tanto trovare altre persone che si trovano nel mio stato per sollevarci vicendevolmente da questo peso.

◆ ❖ ◆

Antonio Sabino
per la sua Madre Gianna
Italy

The English version of this story is in Chapter 2.

Salve, scrivo questa storia a nome di mia madre, la quale non è molto pratica nell'uso del computer. Dunque la malattia venne diagnosticata nel mese di maggio 1998, ma i sintomi erano presenti già molto tempo prima. I primi disturbi si manifestarono alle mani, le quali non avevano più la stessa elasticità, ma cominciarono a diventare bianche, fredde, e sopratutto rigide nei movimenti. Poi la malattia si è estesa in altre parti del corpo, sempre a livello cutaneo con la formazione di macchie e di indurimento della pelle stessa. Successivamente si evidenziarono altre manifestazioni classiche della malattia, tra cui un'esofagite da reflusso gastrico e dolori diffusi che hanno portato ad un ridimensionamento dell'alimentazione e all'assunzione di numerosi farmaci, tra cui cortisonici.

Attualmente mia madre è seguita presso la Clinica Universitaria di Padova, reparto di Reumatologia. Oltre a tutti i classici sintomi della malattia, ora si sono aggiunti anche problemi renali, sempre dovuti alla sclerodermia. Soffre inoltre di ricorrenti episodi di reflusso gastrico prevalentemente notturni che le provocano dolori atroci e di febbre con difficoltà respiratorie, nonchè dI un notevole senso dI gonfiore addominale molto intenso. E' presente inoltre un indurimento della pelle tale che quasi non si riesce a farle nemmeno un prelievo, insieme a mancanza delle forze e spossatezza generale.

A questo punto termino anche perchè forse non riesco ad essere molto preciso, comunque in meno di due anni la vita di mia madre è totalmente cambiata in modo peggiore ma veramente peggiore. Poi leggendo le lettere di altre persone da voi pubblicate, ho riscontrato che i sintomi e relativi farmaci sono gli stessi.

Pertanto se qualcuno di voi avesse voglia di comunicare con lei per un eventuale confronto o solo dialogo nell'intento di migliorare la situazione di coloro che si trovano a dover combattere questa strana ma brutta malattia, vi sarei grato se vi metteste in contatto. Speriamo nella possibilità di avere un colloquio-confronto che possa servirci a vicenda nel superare i problemi creati dalla stessa malattia e dai rispettivi farmaci. Grazie dell'attenzione. Auguro a tutte le persone affette da sclerodermia di riuscire a vivere in maniera decente senza dover sopportare le sofferenze atroci e quello che comporta purtroppo la stessa malattia.

◆ ❖ ◆

Arianna Balduino
Italy

The English version of this story is in Chapter 3.

Mi chiamo Arianna e sono una ragazza di ventisei anni. Nel settembre del 2000 mi è stata finalmente diagnosticata una forma di sclerosi sistemica progressiva, ma tutto era cominciato ben tre anni prima con l'improvviso sbiancamento di un dito, mentre passeggiavo per le vie del centro con le mie compagne dell'università.

Quando mi sono rivolta al mio medico di famiglia, per questo strano fenomeno, mi sono sentita semplicemente rispondere che dovevo mettere i guanti perchè fuori fa freddo!

Dopo alcuni mesi anche altre dita sono state coinvolte da questo fenomeno a cui si associava anche dolore. Niente. Nessuno ha saputo dirmi cosa fosse!

Nell'aprile del 2000, all'improvviso, ho cominciato ad avvertire una sensazione di rigidità diffusa, non riuscivo più a piegarmi per svolgere le usuali faccende domestiche, avevo le caviglie sempre gonfie e le mani cominciavano a deformarsi ed a gonfiarsi. Mia madre notava un certo cambiamento nella mia fisionomia: il naso si affilava e la bocca diventava sempre più stretta.

Sono arrivata a non potermi più alzare da una sedia senza aggrapparmi a qualcosa per tirarmi su.

Ero umiliata! Ma come era possibile che una ragazza di ventiquattro anni avesse l'energia di un'ottantenne? Il mio dottore mi ha detto che forse avevo l'artrite reumatoide senza neanche farmi fare delle analisi.

Tutto è cambiato dopo l'incontro del mio attuale reumatologo che, soltanto guardandomi in faccia, ha compreso la causa delle mie sofferenze. Adesso prendo tanti di quei farmaci che non si contano e faccio fisioterapia; ho conosciuto delle persone meravigliose (i medici dell'ospedale, le infermiere e il fisioterapista, gli altri pazienti del Day Hospital).

Purtroppo tutto questo non è ancora sufficiente poichè la malattia non si arresta, anzi avanza inesorabilmente.

Il mese scorso il mio reumatologo mi ha detto che ho un'infiammazione ai polmoni e che, se non voglio finire in ossigenoterapia, devo iniziare una nuova cura con la ciclofosfamide, che non è priva di pesantissimi effetti collaterali sulle ovaie.Mi è cascato il mondo addosso. Io avevo ancora una speranza di vivere una vita normale, di sposarmi e di avere dei figli!

Forse sono stata un po' presuntuosa, ma adesso ripensandoci quello che voglio è lottare contro questa malattia per impedirle di battermi.

Spero di non avervi annoiato troppo. Vi voglio bene!

Flora Savini
Italy

The English version of this story is in Chapter 3.

Sono una ragazza di ventitre anni e nell' Agosto di quest'anno (1999), dopo un ricovero presso l'Arcispedale Sant'Anna di Ferrara, mi hanno diagnosticato sclerosi sistemica. Soffro inoltre di asma allergico da circa vent'anni.

Attualmente presento acrocianosi alle mani con dita scure e notevole perdita della forza. La funzione respiratoria attualmente è sotto controllo.

Premetto che prima di arrivare a questa diagnosi ho consultato molti medici senza risultati soddisfacenti e con elevate spese.

Vorrei riuscire a conoscere molto meglio gli aspetti della mia malattia con i danni che può provocarmi per poter dare una riposta ai miei dubbi, del tipo "Potrò avere una vita normale?"

Voglio incoraggiare tutte le persone, che come me sono affette da sclerodermia, affinchè riescano a combattere questa malattia.

Ringrazio per questo spazio, che mi è stato dedicato, perchè ho potuto raccontare la mia esperienza e parlare della mia malattia.

◆ ❖ ◆

Giòvanna (Giò) Leonardo
Italy

The English version of this story is in Chapter 3.

Sono affetta da sclerodermia dal 1990. Attualmente assumo terapia con nifedipina, cortisone, aspirina, Calcio e per dieci mesi l'anno vengo sottoposta ad un ciclo di tre giorni al mese di Iloprost (prostaciclina), che devo dire mi ha aiutato molto.

Bisogna essere costanti e non abbassare mai la guardia. Ringrazio tutte quelle persone che mi aiutano ogni giorno a svolgere gli atti quotidiani della vita.

Rouge
Italy

The English version of this story is in Chapter 3.

Ho trentacinque anni e fino a due anni fa pensavo di soffrire solo del fenomeno di Raynaud, ma poi, dopo la comparsa di piccole ulcere sulle dita delle mani ho fatto degli esami immunologici che hanno portato alla diagnosi di Sclerodermia Limitata. Attualmente il mio stato è quello di aver perso un pò di elasticità alle dita e di avere qualche rughetta intorno alla bocca.

Sto prendendo diversi medicinali. Sono anche in cura da un omeopata che mi sta dando dei rimedi per "disintossicarmi" e che mi ha anche mandato dal dentista per farmi togliere l'amalgama (otturazioni con il mercurio) dai denti perchè questa potrebbe incidere con la malattia. Sto anche facendo una dieta: non mangio più pasta e pane se non quella integrale. Io penso che facendoci aiutare dai medici tradizionali e da quelli alternativi la nostra vita possa migliorare notevolmente.

Valeria Macali
Italy

The English version of this story is in Chapter 3.

Sono una ragazza di ventuno anni e, all'età di nove anni, mi è stata diagnosticata la sclerosi sistemica. Da allora sono in cura presso il Policlinico A.Gemelli di Roma. Necessito di uno o due ricoveri l'anno per fare tutti gli esami di routine e per essere sottoposta a varie terapie oltre a svariate creme per il corpo.

Attualmente la mia situazione è la seguente: perdita dell'elasticità della pelle del viso, delle mani e degli avambracci, ridotta motilità esofagea, reflusso gastro-esofageo, gastrite cronica e marcata compromissione circolatoria delle estremità delle dita delle mani e dei piedi.

Nell'Aprile 1999 ho iniziato una nuova cura con vasodilatatori per via endovenosa (prostaciclina) ad intervalli di 3 mesi l'uno dall'altro, per ogni due mesi che sto a casa trascorro circa un mese in ospedale. Non ho voglia di spiegare quanto mi sia costata questa malattia in termini di sofferenza fisica e morale e quanto essa sia riuscita a condizionare la mia vita, non riuscirei a trovare le parole adatte.

Vorrei riuscire a conoscere tutte le terapie possibili per questa malattia, tutti i centri che si occupano di essa (in Italia e all'estero), nonchè tutti gli esami necessari per accorgersi prontamente dei danni che potrebbe provocare. Mi farebbe anche molto piacere sapere se esiste qualche centro, possibilmente non troppo lontano da Roma, dove poter fare un'adeguata fisioterapia per il viso e le mani, visto che mi rimane faticoso anche arrotolare gli spaghetti e che non riesco neanche a ridere perchè mi vengono subito i crampi alle guance.

Vorrei anche dire che in questo mio cammino hanno avuto un ruolo fondamentale i miei amici che non hanno permesso che mi sentissi sola neanche per un istante. Senza la loro presenza e il loro sostegno non sarei mai riuscita a superare le umiliazioni e le sofferenze dei miei ultimi ricoveri. A tutte le persone che hanno la mia stessa malattia vorrei dire una cosa: non permettete che la sclerodermia, insieme al vostro corpo logori anche il vostro cuore. A voi tutti un grazie sincero per l'aiuto che potete darmi.

◆ ❖ ◆

Alex
Italy

The English version of this story is in Chapter 6.

Sono una donna di trentaquattro anni e sono affetta da sclerodermia localizzata da circa vent'anni.

La malattia inizialmente si è manifestata con una macchia molto piccola sulla coscia destra che sembrava essere un ematoma. In seguito, la lesione ha cambiato aspetto più volte e si è estesa su tutta la gamba. Inoltre è apparsa anche una piccola macchia sul viso che quasi certamente è un'altra manifestazione della stessa malattia.

Ho interpellato diversi specialisti, quasi tutti concordi sulla diagnosi e sull'impossibilità di eseguire una terapia ad hoc, spiegandomi che non si conosce ancora l'origine vera e propria della malattia e quindi la cura.

Mi hanno suggerito di effettuare diverse terapie che non hanno dato grossi risultati se non quello di ammorbidire la pelle.

Ho fatto una serie di accertamenti immunologici (tra cui gli anticorpi anti-nucleo) per verificare la possibilità che si trattasse di una forma sistemica. Fortunatamente questi esami sono risultati tutti negativi. Adesso, dopo aver letto le informazioni di questo sito, non sono più sicura che questi risultati escludano totalmente la forma più grave di questa malattia. Per la cronaca: sono anche affetta da morbo celiaco. Grazie.

Franco Pilone
Italy

The English version of this story is in Chapter 7.

Ciao a tutti, mi chiamo Franco, ho cinquantasette anni e tre anni fa mi è stata diagnosticata la sindrome di Sjögren, ma in realtà sono quasi trent'anni che ne soffro. Prima della diagnosi il mio medico mi ha fatto fare tantissimi esami particolari, dopodiché ha tratto le proprie conclusioni.

Dieci anni fa mi sono ammalato di pericardite essudativa autoimmune: ho sofferto tanto! Ho preso diversi farmaci fra cui il cortisone, ma il problema non si risolveva. Tre anni fa sono stato sottoposto ad una pericardiectomia ed ho sperato che tutto si fosse risolto; invece continuo ad avere dolori toracici e non posso fare a meno di assumere il cortisone.

Ho subito l'asportazione della ghiandola salivare, soffro di artrite reumatoide ed adesso ho seri problemi agli occhi; infatti la scarsa lacrimazione ha avuto come conseguenza un'infiammazione delle cornee. Ho forti dolori con disturbi intestinali, sempre dovuti alla sindrome di Sjögren. Mi affatico spesso quando cammino un po' veloce e ad ogni sforzo.

Attualmente sono in cura da un immunologo presso l'ospedale "Niguarda" di Milano ed assumo varie terapie ed antidolorifici al bisogno. Anche avendo tutti questi problemi vado ugualmente avanti con la speranza che si possa trovare una cura per questa malattia.

V. O.
Italy

The English version of this story is in Chapter 7.

Sono una ragazza di trent'anni e da tre sono affetta da Sindrome di Sjögren con alta positività per anticorpi anti-SSA.

Sono in trattamento con cortisonici e, da circa un anno, è comparso un picco monoclonale nel sangue. Continuo a fare lo stesso trattamento con cortisone anche se recentemente, a seguito dello stress, ho avuto una riacutizzazione dei sintomi con dolore alla parotide di destra risolti dopo aver aumentato il dosaggio dello steroide.

Sono molto preoccupata per il mio stato, sono iscritta all'associazione senza grande aiuto, vorrei mettermi in contatto con altri colleghi (sono infatti un medico) che mi possano aiutare e dare soprattutto la loro esperienza.

Vorrei avere inoltre informazioni circa la possibilità di avere una gravidanza e per quanto riguarda lo sviluppo di neoplasie.

CHAPTER 11

Polski (Polish)

Anna
Poland

The English version of this story is in Chapter 6.

Moja historia zaczęła się dokładnie dziewięć lat temu. Dnia 11.08.93 roku w wieku 18 lat zostałam przyjęta do szpitala z powodu bólów dużych stawów kończyn górnych i dolnych z ograniczeniem ruchomości, utrzymujących się od 6-ciu miesięcy. Na podstawie obrazu klinicznego i badań dodatkowych rozpoznano młodzieńczą postać RZS. Celem dalszych badań diagnostycznych i leczenia specjalistycznego zostałam przekazana na oddział Reumatologiczny. Byłam w ciężkim stanie. Badaniem fizykalnym stwierdzono ogólne wyniszczenie, bladość powłok skórnych, tachykardię, powiększoną wątrobę, przykurcze w stawach łokciowych, ograniczenie ruchomości w stawach barkowych i kolanowych, bolesność i ograniczenie ruchomości nadgarstków, bolesność w stawach sródstopno-palcowych. W badaniach laboratoryjnych stwierdzono znacznie przyspieszone OB, anemię, obniżony poziom żelaza, erytrocyturię. Ponadto w badaniach dodatkowych wykazano dodatni test LE oraz obecność przeciwciał przeciwjądrowych o wysokim mianie.

Całość obrazu klinicznego oraz badań dodatkowych pozwoliła na wstępne rozpoznanie tocznia rumieniowatego układowego. W trakcie hospitalizacji wystąpiły zaburzenia ukrwienia obwodowego, manifestujące się marmurkowym zabarwieniem, ochłodzeniem i stwardnieniem skóry kończyny dolnej prawej, szczególnie w zakresie powierzchni bocznej grzbietu stopy. Wystapienie powyżej opisywanych zmian nasunęło podejrzenie mieszanej postaci kolagenozy. Po trzech miesiącach w stanie zadawalającym zostałam wypisana do domu z zaleceniem systematycznej kontroli w poradni Reumatologicznej i pobierania leków, miedzy innymi sterydów.

To były początki rozpoznawania mojej choroby. Wtedy nie zdawałam sobie sprawy z powagi tych chorób i do czego mogą doprowadzić człowieka. Żyłam dalej, brałam leki i jednocześnie patrzyłam, jak jedna z tych chorób zabiera mi ojca. Niszczyła go powoli, zaatakowała mu serce, pewnego dnia zasnął i się nie obudził. Jego śmierć była dla mnie strasznym szokiem. Zostalismy sami ja i moi bracia, z tym że jeden z nich od dwóch lat przebywał za granicą. Mamę straciliśmy, gdy byliśmy jeszcze dziećmi.

Pięć miesięcy później na prawej nodze i prawej ręce zaczęła twardnieć skóra. W związku z tym zgłosiłam się ponownie do szpitala, w którym przebywałam wcześniej. Rozpoznano: Zespół nakładania tocznia układowego i sklerodermii.

Po miesiącu, z uwagi na brak możliwości wykonania specjalistycznych badań i uściślenie rozpoznania, przewieziono mnie do Kliniki Dermatologicznej.

W tej klinice rozpoznano: Sclerodermia linearis gravis (linijna), Polyarthritis rheumatoidea ad exploratione, wreszcie twardzinę linijną o ciężkim przebiegu. Zainteresowałam się w końcu, co to jest ta sklerodermia. Podejrzewałam, że jest to groźna choroba i chciałam dowiedzieć się o niej czegoś więcej. W klinice poznałam trzy pacjentki cierpiące na twardzinę. Wyglądały strasznie, przypominały mumie. Jedna z nich miała skrócone palce u rąk, na twarzy skórę naciągniętą, wydawałoby się, jakby każde ich słowo czy mimika sprawiały im ból. Bałam się, że widzę siebie w przyszłości, że mnie czeka to samo. Co czuje młoda dziewczyna widząc skutki choroby, którą właśnie lekarze u niej stwierdzili? No cóż, czuje wielki lęk, strach przed śmiercią, że może nadejść zbyt szybko, a po drodze przysporzyć jej wiele cierpień. Czuje wielki żal, że właśnie ją to spotkało. Wszystkie plany na przyszłość widzi w czarnych kolorach. Zamyka się w sobie i czeka, co będzie dalej. Tak do końca nie da się opisać tego co czuje; ten, kto tego nie przeżył, nie jest w stanie pojąć, co przeżywa chory człowiek.

W szpitalu jedna z pacjentek pożyczyła mi książkę, w której była opisana sklerodermia. Gdy ją przeczytałam, nie mogłam uwierzyć, że właśnie mnie to spotkało. Zadawałam sobie pytanie: "dlaczego?", na które nie znałam odpowiedzi. Wiedziałam tylko tyle, że twardzina linijna nie jest taka groźna, że zajmuje tylko skórę, nigdy nie atakuje organów wewnętrznych, jedynie co może okaleczyć człowieka. Ja do końca nie wiedziałam, ktorą z nich mam, dlatego okropnie się bałam, modliłam się o jej łagodniejszą postać. W moim przypadku lekarze zastanawiali się, czy moje schorzenie ma charakter zespołu nakładania, czy jest to twardzina linijna o ciężkim przebiegu. W związku z tym z Kliniki Dermatologicznej zostałam przekazana na oddział Internistyczno-Reumatologiczny.

Po dwóch tygodniach pobytu w tym szpitalu postawiono ostateczną diagnozę: MCTD(mieszana choroba tkanki łącznej). Czyli z tego co zrozumiałam, nie był to toczeń rumieniowaty układowy, ani nie była to twardzina linijna o ciężkim przebiegu. Sama nie wiedziałam, która z tych chorób jest gorsza, nie wiedziałam w co już wierzyć, w każdym szpitalu inna diagnoza, ale cóż, teraz już wiem, że w tych chorobach kolagenowych nie łatwo ją ustalić.

Po wyjściu ze szpitala w 1994r. załamałam się, nie wiedziałam co mnie czeka. Mój brat, który ze mną mieszkał, wyjechał za granicę. Zostałam sama ze swoją chorobą, której nienawidziłam i nie chciałam w nią uwierzyć. Przypominały mi jednak o niej bóle stawów, jak również moja twardniejąca noga i ręka. Nie wierzyłam w to, że mam jakiekolwiek szanse na normalne życie, dla mnie przyszłość przestała istnieć. Przestałam się leczyć, a zaczęłam pić alkohol, nie zależało mi na niczym. Piłam, a gdy bolały mnie kości, zażywałam sterydy (Encorton). Po jakimś czasie moja noga zaczęła wyglądać jak poparzona, zanikły mięśnie i zrobiła się twarda jak kamień, szczególnie na skórze kończyny dolnej prawej. Wtedy zaczęłam pić więcej, żeby zapomnieć. Najgorszą porą roku było dla mnie lato. Musiałam pocić się w długich spodniach i w bluzkach z długimi rękawami. Idąc przez miasto i widząc uśmiechniętych, lekko ubranych ludzi czułam żal, że ja już do nich nie należę. Więc najlepszym moim przyjacielem stał się alkohol.

Po dwoch - trzech miesiącach moje dolegliwości reumatyczne ustąpiły, pojawiały się od czasu do czasu. Zdążyłam się do nich przyzwyczaić. Od 1994 do 1998r. moje życie nie miało sensu, żyłam z dnia na dzień i zastanawiałam się, jak je zakończyc (miałam myśli samobójcze). Aż do dnia, kiedy dowiedziałam się, że jestem w ciąży. Wtedy wróciła mi ochota do życia, poczułam się jak nowonarodzona. Byłam taka szczęśliwa, a zarazem bałam się o stan dziecka, tyle lat się nie leczyłam. O dziwo alkohol nie dokonał żadnych szkodliwych zmian w moim organiźmie. Choroba jakby stanęła, odeszła ode mnie, ale nie na długo. Nigdy nie myślałam, że kiedykolwiek przy tej chorobie będę mogła mieć dziecko. Bardzo pragnęłam mieć dziewczynkę. W czasie ciąży choroba nie dawała o sobie znaku. Czułam się jak normalna zdrowa kobieta, która nosi w sobie życie. Myślę, że za szybko poddałam się chorobie, straciłam nadzieję, która przy leczeniu jest bardzo potrzebna. Nie dałam sobie szansy na normalne życie, wprowadzałam się w stan samozniszczenia. Dopiero ciąża wszystko odmieniła, to był początek rozpoczęcia przeze mnie normalnego życia i chęć walki z chorobą. Przez całe dziewięć miesięcy dbałam o siebie i ciążę, wszystko przebiegało w jak najlepszym porządku, nie dopuszczałam do siebie mysli, że coś może być nie tak, po prostu wierzyłam w to, że dziecko da mi szczęście, a wiara może zdziałać cuda. Wreszcie nadszedł dzień rozwiązania. Urodziłam zdrową dziewczynkę. To był najszczęśliwszy dzień w moim życiu. Teraz miałam dla kogo żyć.

W 1998 roku na Sylwestra poznałam mężczyznę, w którym się zakochałam z wzajemnością. On także odmienił moje życie. Kilkanaście miesięcy później moja choroba dała o sobie znać, położyła mnie na łopatki. Nie mogłam podnieść się z łóżka. Wylądowałam w szpitalu. Po dwutygodniowym pobycie zostałam wypisana do domu, ale tym razem postanowiłam się leczyć, bo miałam już dla kogo. W rok później wyszłam za mąż, zamieszkaliśmy we trójkę. Moj mąż zaakceptował mnie taką jaką jestem. Uświadomiłam sobie, że wygląd zewnętrzny człowieka nie jest najważniejszy, liczy się rodzina i miłość, bez której czy jesteś zdrowy czy chory ciężko jest żyć. Dzięki niemu zaakceptowałam sama siebie.

W 2001r. w Klinice Dermatologicznej rozpoznano: wypaloną sklerodermię prawej ręki i prawej nogi, które wymagają tylko higienicznego trybu życia, intensywnej higieny skóry. Obecnie przechodzę terapię w związku z problemami reumatycznymi. Jestem szczęśliwa, że moje życie, pomimo wielu złych przeżyć, zrezygnowań, nabrało sensu. Doszłam do wniosku, że nie warto rezygnować z niego, nawet w tych najtrudniejszych chwilach, trzeba je przetrwać i wierzyć że będzie lepiej. Gdybym w to nie wierzyła, nie pisałabym teraz mojej historii. Moja córeczka obecnie ma 3,5 r. A my z mężem pod kontrolą lekarzy planujemy dziecko. Teraz już wiem, że nie jest to choroba dziedziczna, zdrowa matka może urodzić chore dziecko, tak samo jak i chora matka może urodzić zdrowe dziecko, tak jak to było w moim przypadku.

CHAPTER 12

Romana (Romanian)

Krista Lurtz
Romania

The English version of this story is in Chapter 8.

Nu este prea usor, sa incepi sa-ti scri propria istorie, in asemenea situatie.

De ce? Pentru ca habar nu am daca sa scriu despre Krista de acum citiva ani, sau Krista cea de acum. Da, sunt tot eu. Dar sub o alta forma fizica.

Cind vorbim despre cursul vietii, putem spune ca viata pleaca din copilarie, urci pe culmea ei, si dupa, incepi si coborirea, fireste. Normal, coborirea se face lin, placut, cu satisfactiile ce le-ai adunat pe culme.

Eu ce sa spun? Am ajuns pe culme, si nici nu am ajuns bine, ca ma trezesc luind-o de vale cu o viteza fantastica! Normal, nu spre copilarie.

Si totusi, acum citiva ani, acasa fiind, (in zona Fagarasului) cu muntele la capatii, este normal, ca am fost si inca mai sunt indragostita de el.

Muntele, padurea, tot ce se cheama natura, au facut parte din viata mea. Pina si pesterile, prin care m-am tirit citiva ani, culegind oase de "ursus peleus".

S-a intimplat sa plec din tara. Am ajuns aici, in Qatar, in mijlocul desher-tului, unde peisajul ma darima. Departe de casa, cu dor de tot ce inseamna casa si cei dragi, m-am trezit intr-o buna zi, ca urcind un etaj, sint atit de stoarsa de energie, incit sa fiu nevoita sa ma asez pe scara, sa ma odihnesc. (Nu era nici Omul, nici Moldoveanul. Si nici macar platoul Bucegilor. Erau amaritele de scari din casa.)

Nu mi-au placut niciodata cabinetele medicale, dar de data asta, sim-team ca ceva nu e in regula.

Tot acum citiva ani, am trecut printr-o interventie chirurgicala, la co-loana (hernie de disc). Durerile ramase dupa, le-am pus pe seama acestui fapt, doar ca sa nu ma gindesc la altele.

Ajunsa in cabinetul unui medic de aici, dupa doua ore de explicat ceea ce mi se intimpla (pe linga slabiciune, incepusem sa am tot felul de "arsuri" ale pielii, furnicaturi, spasme musculare, ca si cum, tot corpul meu trecuse la o activitate necunoscuta mie, dar toata ziua, se intimpla ceva.)

Aspectul meu exterior, nu arata in nici un fel, ca as fi bolnava, si s-ar putea spune ca arat "bine" in postura unei femei la 30 de ani. De aici urmarea: medicul se uita la mine, de parca toate cite ii spuneam, sint doar urmarea unei imaginatii bogate. Mi s-a recoltat singe, iar a doua zi, rezultatul a fost:

"Doamna imi pare rau sa va spun ca sinteti perfect sanatoasa!"(analizele medicale, care se fac de rutina asa indicau. Si eu care speram o anemie, o lipsa de calciu, sau ceva!)

Un an mai tirziu, (renuntasem la ideea sa mai merg la medic), simteam ca lucrurile merg din ce in ce mai prost. Incepusem sa pierd uneori controlul reflexelor, lipsa de concentrare, pierderi de memorie, si multe alte noi senzatii. Am repetat experienta medicala, cu acelasi rezultat. Diferenta: am mers la o clinica particulara, si am platit.

De data asta, am insistat, si printr-un prieten, am ajuns la un ortoped. Dupa un consult sumar, diagnostic provizoriu: fibromialgie, suspect lupus. Teama? Mai mult decit teama!

Intimplator, despre lupus, auzisem, si cunoasteam in mare, forma care ataca pielea fetei. Despre fibromialgie, nu stiam nimic. Acasa, conectata la internet, am inceput sa caut, sa aflu, sa stiu. Cele aflate, nu erau deloc incurajatoare. A fost prima data cind am realizat ca ma aflu in teritoriu bolilor incurabile. (Cind am facut greseala sa calc acolo? - nu stiu.)

Soc? Da. Socata, speriata, ingrozita, disperata, toate starile astea m-au napadit dintr-o data. Stiam ca va urma o perioada in care lacrimile vor fi in ochii mei ca la ele acasa. Stiam ca urma sa strabat un drum, anevoios, si mai stiam ca cei din jur, nu ma vor putea ajuta prea mult, in legatura cu ceea ce simteam.

Nu am mai vrut decit sa ma intorc in tara, sa incep acolo greul: teste medicale. Speram ca acasa pot gasi medici care sa ma ajute. Si am gasit.

Cind multi dintre romani pleaca din tara sa caute medici, eu m-am intors in tara. In primul rind simteam nevoia sa vorbesc in propria mea limba, si sa aud la fel.

Prietenii prietenilor, m-au ajutat. Ajunsa la Tg. Mures, Nicu Racheru, (caruia ii multumesc foarte mult), m-a ajutat si dupa 2 saptamini de cautare, am poposit la clinica Nr.2.

A-nceput apoi, greul. Si zile intregi, scurgindu-se la nesfirsit cu teama, in asteptarea unui diagnostic, care nu mai venea. Teste, peste teste, intre Tg.Mures si Cluj, teste noi, teste repetate, radiografii, tot felul de minuni medicale, care nu se mai terminau. Dupa 2 luni, obosita, fara sa ajungem la un rezultat clar, am hotarit sa iau o pauza. Sa mai dam timp bolii sa se faca vazuta mai bine.

Aici, m-a ajutat foarte mult, psihic, faptul ca deja citisem mult despre asemenea boli, si stiam, cit de greu se face diagnosticarea, stiam ca poate dura luni, ani, sau ca pot sa traiesc toata viata nestiind exact numele bolii. Asta nu facea lucrurile mai usoare, dar ma ajuta sa inteleg, si cu timpul sa accept situatia.

In toamna, dupa ce intre timp aparusera citeva crize de dureri infioratoare, m-am intors in tara, la medicii mei. Si iar a inceput virtejul testelor. Dar, acum aveam avantajul ca prin multe trecusem, si erau eliminate.

Toata perioada, a fost un razboi al nervilor. Ma consider norocoasa, pentru ca am avut alaturi, prieteni dragi. In primul rind, buna si batrina mea prietena Lili, care a fost linga mine, aproape zilnic. Si Nicu, cel care, nu numai ca ma gazduia, dar ma mai si urca precum sacul de cartofi, la etajul 4 (daca statea asa sus!?)

Tg. Mures- Cluj-Tg. Mures. Laboratoare, medici, seringi, teste, biopsie. In final, diagnostic: Scleroderma, Vasculita, Polimiozita. Frumoasa colectie de boli autoimune, incurabile.

DE CE EU? (intrebare pentru univers) M-am trezit cazind in hau, in necunoscut, trebuind cumva, la 30 de ani, sa incep sa invat sa traiesc. Nu e usor. Nu e usor deloc. Dar, atit cit pot, am sa incerc sa lupt, intr-un fel sau altul. Iar prin munca mea, la aceasta pagina, as dori sa pot sa ajut pe cei ca mine.

"Nu lupt pentru a trai, ci traiesc pentru a lupta!"

Conclusion
by Shelley L. Ensz

Voices of Scleroderma has shown us the height of courage of those who have lived, and died, with scleroderma and related illnesses. They have given us all the gift of their stories in the hopes of making it easier for those who follow in our footsteps.

As you can see, not even one hundred stories begin to tell the saga of scleroderma, because it is so vastly different in every case with its onset, severity, symptoms, course and outcome. And not even one thousand stories would clearly expose the dire and urgent need for more scleroderma information, support, awareness, and research throughout the world.

Yet, at the same time, every single story does tell the story of scleroderma; every single story does expose the need for a cure; every single story offers its own ray of hope, its own form of support.

Have you found solace and strength in this book and courage to continue your battle with illness or caregiving? Have you wept with grief or compassion from the stories of those who are suffering, or who have died? Have their plainly detailed struggles whisked you away to seldom visited corners of your soul, changed the way you feel about your life, your health, your loved ones, your values, the sanctity of life, the importance of cherishing each and every moment we are gifted?

Whether or not you or a loved one has scleroderma or related illnesses, if you feel warmed by compassion and stirred to action by our plight of the "disease that turns people to stone," we invite you to continue to support the cause of scleroderma in your community and throughout the world. The world desperately needs your gifts time, talent, and contributions to provide more scleroderma information, support and research, worldwide.

By joining our hands together around the world, by committing ourselves to an end to this suffering, someday our voices of scleroderma will be heard around the world! Someday, there will be a cure!

And it will be because you joined us in this worthy cause and left your footprints in the sand.

◆❖◆

Scleroderma Resources

International Scleroderma Network (ISN)

The ISN is a nonprofit, charitable organization that offers worldwide medical, support, and awareness information for scleroderma and related illnesses. See **www.sclero.org**.

Juvenile Scleroderma Network (JSDN)

The JSDN is a nonprofit agency that provides online support and information for juvenile scleroderma. See **www.jsdn.org**.

Scleroderma Clinical Trials Consortium (SCTC)

The SCTC is a charitable, nonprofit organization dedicated to finding better treatment for scleroderma. Over 50 SCTC member institutions worldwide conduct clinical treatment trials for scleroderma, and they publish the Scleroderma Care and Research Journal. See **www.sctc-online.org**.

ISN/SCTC Research Fund

You may support international scleroderma research via the collaborative ISN/SCTC Research Fund, for top notch peer-reviewed international scleroderma research. See **www.sclero.org**.

Scleroderma Webmaster's Association (SWA)

The ISN also manages the Scleroderma Webmaster's Association, which offers the popular free service, Scleroderma Sites to Surf! Get your group or website listed today! See **www.sclero.org**.

Scleroderma from A to Z Web Site

The ISN operates Scleroderma from A to Z where all the stories in this book were first published. It features hundreds of pages of top notch medical information and support, in many languages. See **www.sclero.org**.

◆ ❖ ◆

Glossary of Medical Terms

A

acid reflux

A burning discomfort behind the lower part of the sternum usually related tospasm of the lower end of the esophagus or of the upper part of the stomachoften in association with gastroesophageal reflux. *See also: heartburn*

allopathy

A system of medical practice that aims to combat disease by use of remedies producing effects different from or incompatible with those produced by the special disease treated.[1]

alopecia

Hair loss or baldness.

alternative medicine

Any of various systems of healing or treating disease (as homeopathy, chiropractic, naturopathy, Ayurveda, or faith healing) that are not included in the traditional curricula taught in medical schools of the U.S. and Britain.[1]

alveoli

Tiny air sacs located at the very ends of the bronchioles within the lungs where the exchange of gases occur between the blood and the air.

amputation

Removal of part or all of a body part enclosed by skin.

ANA *See antinuclear antibodies.*

ankylosing spondylitis

A type of arthritis that affects the spine.

antibody

A special protein produced by the body's immune system that recognizes and helps fight infectious agents and other foreign substances that invade the body.

anxiety

An abnormal and overwhelming sense of apprehension and fear often marked by physiological signs such as sweating, tension and increased pulse.

antinuclear antibodies (ANA)

Antibodies or autoantibodies that react with components and especially DNA of cell nuclei and that tend to occur frequently in connective tissue diseases (as systemic lupus erythematosus, rheumatoid arthritis, and Sjögren's syndrome).

arrhythmias
An alteration in rhythm of the heartbeat either in time or force.[1]

arthritis
Inflammation of a joint. When joints are inflamed they can develop stiffness, warmth, swelling, redness and pain. There are over one hundred types of arthritis.

aspiration pneumonia
Infection of the lungs due to aspiration (the sucking in of food particles or fluids into the lungs).

autoimmune disease
An illness that occurs when the body tissues are attacked by its own immune system, such as Hashimoto's thyroiditis, polymyositis, rheumatoid arthritis, scleroderma, Sjögren's syndrome, and systemic lupus erythematosus.

B

Barrett's esophagus
Metaplasia of the lower esophagus that is characterized by replacement of squamous epithelium with columnar epithelium, occurs especially as a result of chronic gastoesophageal reflux, and is associated with an increased risk for esophageal carcinoma.[1]

biopsy
The removal and examination of the tissue, cells, or fluids from the living body.[1]

bowel disease, inflammatory
A group of chronic intestinal diseases characterized by inflammation of the bowel, such as ulcerative colitis and Crohn's disease.

C

calcinosis
An abnormal deposit of calcium salts in body tissues, as is seen in some forms of disease, including CREST, which is a form of systemic scleroderma.

carpal tunnel syndrome (CTS)
A condition caused by compression of the median nerve in the carpal tunnel and characterized especially by weakness, pain, and disturbances of sensation in the hand and fingers.

CAT scan
A scan using computerized axial tomography.[1]

cataract
A clouding of the lens of the eye or its surrounding transparent membrane that obstructs the passage of light.[1]

celiac sprue
A chronic hereditary intestinal disorder in which an inability to absorb the gliadin portion of gluten results in the gliadin triggering an immune response that damages the intestinal mucosa.

chilblains
An inflammatory swelling or sore caused by exposure (as in feet or hands) to cold.[1]

cirrhosis
Widespread disruption of normal liver structure by fibrosis and formation of regenerative nodules that is caused by any of various chronic progressive conditions affecting the liver.[1]

clinical depression
Depression of sufficient severity to be brought to the attention of a physician and to require treatment.[1]

collagen
An insoluble fibrous protein of vertebrates that is the chief constituent of the fibrils of connective tissue (as in skin and tendons) and of the organic substance of bones.

connective tissue disease
Any of various diseases or abnormal stats (as rheumatoid arthritis, systemic lupus erythrmatosus, polyarteritis nodosa, rheumatic fever and dermatomyositis) characterized by inflammatory or degenerative changes in connective tissue.[1]

CREST Syndrome
A limited form of systemic scleroderma.

CT scan
A scan using computerized tomography.

D

dehydration
Process of dehydrating; an abnormal depletion of body fluids.

diffuse scleroderma
A form of systemic scleroderma that generally involves widespread skin involvement.

diverticulitis
Inflammation of diverticulum.

dysphagia
Difficulty swallowing.[1]

E

echocardiography
The use of ultrasound to examine and measure the structure and functioning of the heart and to diagnose abnormalities and disease.[1]

eczema
An inflammatory condition of the skin characterized by redness, itching, and oozing vesicular lesions which become scaly, crusted or hardened.[1]

endocrinology
A science dealing with the endocrine glands.[1]

endometriosis
The presence and growth of functioning endometrial tissue in places other than the uterus that often results in severe pain and infertility.[1]

endoscopic retrograde cholangiopancreatography (ERCP)
Radiographic visualization of the pancreatic and biliary ducts by means of endoscopic injection of a contrast medium through the ampulla of Vater.[1]

eosinophilic fasciitis (Shulman's syndrome)
A disease that leads to inflammation and thickening of the skin and a lining tissue under the skin, called fascia, that covers a surface of underlying tissues.

Epstein-Barr virus
A herpes virus that causes infectious mononucleosis and is associated with Burkitt's lymphoma and nasopharyngeal carcinoma.

erythema nodosum
A skin condition characterized by small tender reddened nodules under the skin (as over the shin bones) often accompanied by fever and transitory arthritic pains and commonly considered a manifestation of hypersensitivity.[1]

esophageal
Of, or relating to, the esophagus (throat).

esophagram
A series of x-rays of the esophagus. The x-ray pictures are taken after the patient drinks a solution that coats and outlines the walls of the esophagus. Also called a barium swallow.

ESR
Abbreviation for erythrocyte sedimentation rate.

F

fainting (syncope)
To lose consciousness because of a temporary decrease in the blood supply to the brain.

fibromyalgia
Any of the group of nonarticular rheumatic disorders characterized by pain, tenderness, and stiffness of muscles and associated connective tissue structures.

G

gallbladder
A membranous muscular sac in which bile from the liver is stored.

gallstones
A calculus formed in the gallbladder or biliary passages.

gangrene
Local death of soft tissues due to loss of blood supply.[1]

gastroesophageal reflux
Backward flow of the gastric contents into the esophagus resulting from improper functioning of the sphincter at the lower end of the esophagus.[1]

gastrointestinal (GI)
Of, relating to, or affecting both stomach and intestine.

gastroscope
An instrument for viewing the interior of the stomach.

GERD
Abbreviation for gastroesophageal reflux disease. A highly variable chronic condition that is characterized by periodic episodes of gastro-esophageal reflux usually accompanied by heartburn and that may result in histopathological changes in the esophagus.

Gilbert's disease
A metabolic disorder probably inherited as an autosomal dominant with variable penetrance and characterized by elevated levels of mostly unconjugated serum bilirubin caused especially by defective uptake of bilirubin by the liver.[1]

H

heart failure
A condition in which the heart is unable to pump blood at an adequate rate or in adequate volume.

heartburn
A burning discomfort behind the lower part of the sternum usually related to spasm of the lower end in association with gastroesophageal reflux.

hematoma
A mass of usually clotted blood that forms in a tissue, organ, or body space as a result of a broken blood vessel.[1]

hepatitis C
Inflammation of the liver that is caused by a single-stranded RNA-containing virus, usually transmitted by parenteral means (as injection of an illicit drug, blood transfusion, or exposure to blood or blood products) and that accounts for most cases of non-A, non-B hepatitis.

hernia
A protrusion of an organ or part through connective tissue or through a wall of the cavity in which it is normally enclosed.

hiatal hernia
A hernia in which an anatomical part (as the stomach) protrudes through the esophageal hiatus of the diaphragm.

high blood pressure
Hypertension; abnormally high arterial blood pressure.

Hodgkin's disease (Hodgkin's lymphoma)
A neoplastic disease that is characterized by progressive enlargement of lymph nodes, spleen, and liver and by progressive anemia.

Holter monitor
A portable device that makes a continuous record of electrical activity of the heart and that can be worn by an ambulatory patient during the course of daily activities for the purpose of detecting fleeting episodes of abnormal heart rhythms.[1]

homeopathy

A system of medical practice that treats a disease especially by the administration of minute doses of a remedy that would in healthy persons produce symptoms similar to those of the disease.[1]

hypertension

Also known as high blood pressure; abnormally high arterial blood pressure.

hypothyroidism

Deficient activity of the thyroid gland. A resultant bodily condition characterized by lowered metabolic rate and general loss of vigor.[1]

I

inflammation

A local response to cellular injury that is marked by capillary dilatation, leukocytic infiltration, redness, heat, pain, swelling, and often loss of function and that serves as a mechanism initiating the elimination of noxious agents and of damaged tissue.[1]

interferon

Any of a group of heat-stable soluble basic antiviral glycoproteins of low molecular weight that are produced usually by cells exposed to the action of a virus, sometimes to the action of another intracellular parasite (as bacterium), or experimentally to the action of some chemicals, and that include some used medically as antiviral or antineoplastic agents.[1]

interstitial cystitis (IC)

A chronic idiopathic cystitis (bladder inflammation) characterized by painful inflammation of the subepithelial connective tissue and often accompanied by Hunner's ulcer.

irritable bowel syndrome (IBS)

A chronic functional disorder of the colon that is characterized by the secretion and passage of large amounts of mucus, by constipation alternating with diarrhea, and by cramping abdominal pain.

J

joint

The point of contact between elements of an animal skeleton whether movable or rigidly fixed together with the surrounding and supporting parts (as membranes, tendons, or ligaments).[1]

juvenile scleroderma (JSD)

Any form of scleroderma that afflicts children. The localized forms of scleroderma (such as linear and morphea) are most common in children.

K
kidney cancer
Malignancy of the kidney.

L
lichen sclerosus (LIKE-in skler-O-sus)
A skin disorder similar to morphea scleroderma. It can affect men, women, or children, but is most common in women. It usually occurs on the vulva (the outer genitalia or sex organ) in women, but sometimes develops on the head of the penis in men. Occasionally, lichen sclerosus is seen on other parts of the body, especially the upper body, breasts, and upper arms.

limited scleroderma
A form of systemic scleroderma where the skin involvement is limited to the hands and/or face.

linear scleroderma
A form of localized scleroderma, a line of thickened skin that can affect the bones and muscles underneath it, thus limiting the motion of the affected joints and muscles. It most often occurs in the arms, legs, or forehead, and may occur in more than one area. It is most likely to be on just one side of the body. Linear scleroderma generally onsets in childhood, and is sometimes characterized by the failure of one arm or leg to grow as rapidly as its counterpart.

lithotripsy
Procedure to break a kidney stone into small particles that can be passed in the urine.

localized scleroderma
Scleroderma that affects only the skin and not the internal organs. Types of localized scleroderma include morphea and linear.

lupus
Any of several diseases (as lupus vulgaris or systemic lupus erythematosus) characterized by skin lesions. *See also: systemic lupus erythematosus (SLE)*

Lyme disease
An acute inflammatory disease that is usually characterized initially by the skin lesion erythema migrans and by fatigue, fever, and chills and if left untreated may later manifest itself in cardiac and neurological disorders, joint pain, and arthritis and that is cased by a spirochete of the genus Borrelia transmitted by the bite of a tick.

lymphoma
A usually malignant tumor of lymphoid tissue.[1]

M
migraine
A condition that is marked by recurrent usually unilateral severe headache often accompanied by nausea and vomiting and followed by sleep, that tends to occur in more than one member of a family, and that is of

uncertain origin though attacks appear to be precipitated by dilatation of intracranial blood vessels.[1]

mixed connective tissue disease (MCTD)
A syndrome characterized by symptoms of various rheumatic diseases (as systemic lupus erythematosus, scleroderma and polymyositis) and by concentrations of antibodies to extractable nuclear antigens.

MRI
A procedure in which magnetic resonance imaging is used.[1]

morphea scleroderma
A form of localized scleroderma that affects only the skin, causing skin patches that may be red, brown, white or purplish in appearance.

mucus
A viscid slippery secretion that is usually rich in mucins and is produced by mucous membranes which it moistens and protects.[1]

multiple sclerosis (MS)
A demyelinating disease marked by patches of hardened tissue in the brain or the spinal cord and associated especially with partial or complete paralysis and jerking muscle tremor.

muscle
A body tissue consisting of long cells that contract when stimulated and produce motion.[1]

N

nephrectomy
The surgical removal of a kidney.[1]

neuropathy
An abnormal and usually degenerative state of the nervous system or nerves; also a systemic condition (as muscular atrophy) that stems from a neuropathy.[1]

O

oesophagus
Alternate spelling for esophagus.

osteoarthritis
Arthritis of middle age characterized by degenerative and sometimes hypertrophic changes in the bone and cartilage of one or more joints and a progressive wearing down of apposing joint surfaces with consequent distortion of joint position usually without bony stiffening.[1]

osteomyelitis
An infectious inflammatory disease of bone that is often of bacterial origin and is marked by local death and separation of tissue.[1]

P-Q

palpitations
A rapid pulsation; an abnormally rapid beating of the heart when excited by violent exertion, strong emotion or disease.

pancreatitis
Inflammation of the pancreas.[1]

pemphigus
An autoimmune skin disorder characterized by blistering of the skin and mucous membrane.

peripheral neuropathy
A problem with the functioning of the nerves outside the spinal cord. Syptoms may include numbness, weakness, burning pain (especially at night), and loss of reflexes.

petechiae
Pinpoint flat round red spots under the skin caused by intradermal hemorrhage (bleeding into the skin).

pituitary tumor
A growth that arises in the pituitary gland.

plaque, skin
A localized abnormal patch on a body part or surface and especially on the skin.

pleurisy
Painful and difficult respiration, cough and exudation of fluid or fibrinous material into the pleural cavity.

pneumonia
An infection that occurs when fluid and cells collect in the lungs.

polyp
A projecting mass of swollen and hypertrophied or tumorous membrane.

prostaglandin
Any of various oxygenated unsaturated cyclic fatty acids of animals that have a variety of hormone-like actions (as in controlling blood pressure or smooth muscle contraction).

psoriatic arthritis
A severe form of arthritis accompanied by psoriasis, which is a chronic skin disease characterized by circumscribed red patches covered with white scales.

pulmonary embolism
Embolism of a pulmonary artery or one of its branches.

pulmonary fibrosis
Scarring throughout the lungs which can be caused by many conditions, such as sarcoidosis, hypersensitivity pneumonitis, asbestosis, and certain medications.

pulmonary function test
A test designed to measure how well the lungs are working.

pulmonary hypertension
High blood pressure in the pulmonary arteries.

pulmonologist
A doctor that specializes in lung disorders.

purpura
A hemorrhage area in the surface of the skin.

PUVA
PUVA stands for psoralen and ultraviolet A (UVA) therapy in which the patient is exposed first to psoralens (drugs containing chemicals that react with ultraviolet light to cause darkening of the skin) and then to UVA light.

R

rash
An eruption on the body typically with little or no elevation above the surface.[1]

Raynaud's
A vascular disorder that is marked by recurrent spasm of the capillaries and especially of the fingers and toes upon exposure to cold, that is characterized by pallor, cyanosis, and a redness in succession usually accompanied by pain, and that in severe cases progresses to local gangrene.

reflux, esophageal
A condition wherein stomach contents regurgitate or back up (reflux) into the esophagus (throat).

restless leg syndrome (RLS)
A condition that is characterized by creepy-crawly sensations in the limbs, primary in the legs (but occasionally in the arms and trunk).

rheumatoid arthritis
A usually chronic disease that is considered an autoimmune disease and is characterized by pain, stiffness, inflammation, swelling, and sometimes destruction of joints.

rheumatologist
A specialist in rheumatology, a medical science dealing with rheumatic diseases, which are any of various conditions characterized by inflammation or pain in muscles, joints, or fibrous tissue. Scleroderma is considered to be a rheumatic disease.

rosacea
Acne involving the skin of the nose, forehead, and cheeks that is common in middle age and is characterized by congestion, flushing, telangiectasia, and marked nodular swelling of tissues, especially of the nose. Also called acne rosacea.

rotator cuff
A supporting and strengthening structure of the shoulder joint that is made up of part of its capsule blended with tendons of the subscapularis,

infraspinatus, supraspinatus, and teres minor muscles as they pass to the capsule or across it to insert on the humerus.[1]

rotator cuff disease

Damage to the rotator cuff, a group of four tendons that stabilize the shoulder joint and move the shoulder in various directions.

S

sclerodactyly

Scleroderma of the fingers and toes.[1]

scleroderma

A disease of the connective tissue. There are many different types of scleroderma. Some affect only the skin, while other types also affect the internal organs. *See also:* diffuse scleroderma, linear scleroderma, localized scleroderma, morphea scleroderma, and systemic scleroderma

sedimentation rate

The speed at which red blood cells settle to the bottom of a column of citrated blood measured in millimeters deposited per hour and which is used especially in diagnosing the progress of various abnormal conditions.

seizure

Uncontrolled electrical activity in the brain, which may produce a physical convulsion, minor physical signs, thought disturbances, or a combination of symptoms.

Sjögren's syndrome

A chronic inflammatory autoimmune disease that affects especially older women, that is characterized by dryness of mucous membranes especially of the eyes and mouth and by infiltration of the affected tissues by lymphocytes, and that is often associated with rheumatoid arthritis.[1]

skeletal

Pertaining to the skeleton, the bones of the body which collectively provide the framework for the body.

skin plaque

A plaque is a broad, raised area on the skin. Because it is raised, it can be felt.

sleep apnea

Brief periods of recurrent cessation of breathing during sleep that is caused especially by obstruction of the airway or a disturbance in the brain's respiratory center and is associated especially with excessive daytime sleepiness.[1]

spinal stenosis

A narrowing of the lumbar spinal column that produces pressure on the nerve roots resulting in sciatica and a condition resembling intermittent claudication and that usually occurs in middle or old age.[1]

staph infection

Infection with staphylococcal bacteria.

stem cell transplantation
The use of stem cells as a treatment for cancer or other diseases.

stress
A physical, chemical, or emotional factor that causes bodily or mental tension and may be a factor in disease causation; a state of bodily or mental tension resulting from factors that tend to alter an existent equilibrium.[1]

systemic lupus erythematosus (SLE)
An inflammatory connective tissue disease of unknown cause that occurs chiefly in women and that is characterized especially by fever, skin rash, and arthritis, often by acute hemolytic anemia, by small hemorrhages in the skin and mucous membranes, by inflammation of the pericardium, and in serious cases by involvement of the kidneys and central nervous system.[1]

systemic sclerosis (scleroderma)
The type of scleroderma that can cause damage to skin, blood vessels, and internal organs. Subtypes include CREST, limited and diffuse scleroderma.

T

T cell
Any of several lymphocytes (as a helper T cell) that differentiate in the thymus, possess highly specific cell surface antigen receptors, and include some that control the initiation or suppression of cell-mediated and humoral immunity (as by the regulation of T and B cell maturation and proliferation) and others that lyse antigen-bearing cells.[1]

telangiectasia
An abnormal dilatation of capillary vessels and arterioles that often forms an angioma. (Plural: telangiectasias or telangiectases.)[1]

temporomandibular joint (TMJ)
The diarthrosis between the temporal bone and mandible that includes the condyloid process below separated by an articular disk from the glenoid fossa above and that allow for the opening, closing, protrusion, retraction, and lateral movement of the mandible.[1]

temporomandibular joint syndrome (TMJ syndrome)
A group of symptoms that may include pain in the temporomandibular joint, headache, earache, neck, back, or shoulder pain, limited jaw movement, or a clicking or popping sound in the jaw and that are caused either by dysfunction of the temporomandibular joint (as derangement of the articular disk) or another problem (as spasm of the masticatory muscles) affecting the region of the temporomandibular joint. Also called temporomandibular disorder.[1]

thyroiditis, Hashimoto's
A chronic autoimmune thyroiditis that is characterized by thyroid enlargement, thyroid fibrosis, lymphatic infiltration of thyroid tissue, and the production of antibodies which attack the thyroid. It occurs more often in women than men and increases in frequency of occurrence with age.

thyroid

A large bilobed endocrine gland of craniate vertebrates that arises as a median ventral outgrowth of the pharynx, lies in the anterior base of the neck or anterior ventral part of the thorax, is often accompanied by lateral accessory glands sometimes more or less fused with the main mass, and produces especially the hormones thyroxine and triiodothyronine.

titer

The strength of a solution or the concentration of a substance in solution as determined by titration.[1]

TPN

Total parenteral nutrition, intravenous feeding that provides a patient with fluid and essential nutrients.

tracheostomy

The surgical formation of an opening into the trachea through the neck especially to allow the passage of air.[1]

U

ulceration

The process of becoming ulcerated; state of being ulcerated.[1]

ultrasound

A noninvasive technique involving the formation of a two-dimensional image used for the examination and measurement of internal body structures and the detection of bodily abnormalities.[1]

undifferentiated connective tissue disease (UCTD)

When a person has symptoms of various connective tissue diseases without meeting the full criteria for any one of them, it is often called undifferentiated connective tissue disease.

V-Z

ventilator

Also known as respirator. A mechanical device for maintaining artificial respiration.

vitiligo

A skin disorder manifested by smooth white spots on various parts of the body.[1]

Index

About the Editors

Judith R. Thompson is Chair of the ISN Archive Development Committee and author of three published novels: *The Kiss of Judas*, *A Switch In Time* and *Mind Blindness*. She also collaborates with Shelley Ensz for the ISN's *Voices of Scleroderma* book series.

She resides in New Hampshire. She was diagnosed with CREST/ systemic sclerosis in 1991 and has been on disability since then. Judith attended Dean Junior College in Franklin, Massachusetts. She holds a certificate for successful Hospice Volunteer Training and for Mediation Training.

She participated in a drug research program for scleroderma at the Boston University Medical Center with Dr. Joseph Korn as well as participated in the Scleroderma Family Registry and DNA Repository with NIH, presided over by Dr. Maureen D. Mayes.

Shelley L. Ensz is Founder and President of the nonprofit International Scleroderma Network, the Scleroderma from A to Z website, the Scleroderma Webmaster's Association, and EdinaWebDesign.com. She lives in Minnesota with her marvelous husband Gene, and their delightful Senegal parrot, Webstergirl.

The **International Scleroderma Network (ISN)** is a nonprofit organization that provides scleroderma medical and support information and works to raise awareness of scleroderma throughout the world. We also support international medical research for scleroderma through the ISN/SCTC Research Fund.

The ISN is an outgrowth of the Scleroderma from A to Z website at www.sclero.org, where the personal stories in this book were first published. Our website offers hundreds of pages of scleroderma medical and support information in many languages.

Over five dozen virtual volunteers from around the world operate the ISN website, book series, online support community, medical advisory, translation services, hotline, email support, and newsletter production services. We invite you to become an ISN member, donor and/or volunteer today, to help tackle scleroderma!

ISN Membership and Donation Form

The ISN is a registered 501(c)(3) nonprofit agency based in the USA.
We send acknowledgements for all contributions.

❑ ISN Comprehensive Fund, Tackles Scleroderma on all fronts! Enclosed
is my gift to ISN in the amount of $_____ (U.S. funds) to provide a
powerhouse of scleroderma research, support, education and awareness.

❑ ISN/SCTC Research Only Fund. Enclosed is my gift in the amount of
$_____ for international peer-reviewed scleroderma research.

❑ My donation is in loving memory of: _____

ISN Membership

❑ Email Membership. Enclosed is $25.00 or more (U.S. funds only) for an
annual ISN Email Membership or Renewal (in English) to receive the ISN
Insider Newsletter only by email.

❑ Postal Mail Membership. Enclosed is $35.00 or more (U.S. funds) for an an-
nual ISN Postal Mail Membership or Renewal (in English) to receive the ISN
Insider Newsletter through postal mail.

ISN Voices of Scleroderma Books:

❑ Volume 1: Enclosed is $25 per book (includes shipping) for _____ books.
❑ Volume 2: Enclosed is $25 per book (includes shipping) for _____ books.
❑ Volume 3: Enclosed is $25 per book (includes shipping) for _____ books

Notes:

Your Name (first, last): _____

Address: _____

City: _____ State:_____ ZIP:_____

Country: _____ Phone:_____

Email: _____

Pay by: Total: $_____ (U.S. funds)
❑ Check   Cardholder: _____
❑ Visa   Card #: _____
❑ Mastercard Card Expiration Date: (month/year): _____
❑ AMEX   Verification Number: On the back side of your card,
                  there is a long number. What are the last four digits? _____

Please mail this form with payment made out to:
International Scleroderma Network
7455 France Ave So #266
Edina, MN 55435 USA

◆ ❖ ◆

1027474

Made in the USA